Essentials of Mental Health Care

Planning and Interventions

BARBARA B. BAUER, R.N., M.S.N.

Educational Services Director,
Brown County Mental Health Center
Green Bay, Wisconsin

SIGNE S. HILL, R.N., B.S.N., M.A.

Instructor, Practical Nurse Program,
Northeast Wisconsin Technical Institute,
Green Bay, Wisconsin

1986

W. B. SAUNDERS COMPANY

Philadelphia, London, Toronto, Mexico City, Rio de Janeiro, Sydney, Tokyo, Hong Kong

W. B. SAUNDERS COMPANY
Harcourt Brace Jovanovich, Inc.

The Curtis Center
Independence Square West
Philadelphia, PA 19106

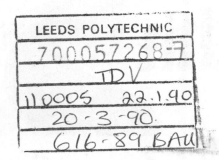

Library of Congress Cataloging-in-Publication Data

Bauer, Barbara B.
  Essentials of mental health care.

  Includes index.
  1. Psychiatric nursing.   2. Mental health planning.
1. Hill, Signe. II. Title. (DNI.M: 1. Mental
Disorders—nursing. 2. Mental Disorders—therapy—
nurses' instruction. 3. Patient Care Planning — methods—
nurses' instruction. WY 160 B344e]
RC440.B35   1986   616.89'0068   85-19617
ISBN 0-7216-1367-5

Editor: Ilze Rader

Developmental Editor: Alan Sorkowitz

Production Manager: Frank Polizzano

Essentials of Mental Health Care—*Planning and Interventions* ISBN   0-7216-1367-5

Last digit is the print number: 9   8   7   6   5

DEDICATION

To our clients, who have enhanced
our learning and helped us
separate the wheat from the chaff.

PREFACE

Most of the positive movement in mental health care has occurred in the past four decades. With a significant number of changes occurring in a comparatively short time, many health providers have entered the field. The providers include nurses from all types of programs, social workers, psychologists, psychiatrists, mental health counselors, psychiatric technicians, occupational therapists, clinical therapists, students at any level, and volunteers. Because of our extensive involvement in mental health as practitioners and educators, we have observed some very definite needs in the health providers' care of the mentally ill client. The greatest difficulty lies in *defining specific problem behaviors, planning realistic approaches related to the problems, and writing measurable, time-limited goals.* This was the initial motivation for writing this book. We believe that it will be a useful reference in planning care.

The book is divided into six units, each unit having a particular focus. Unit I focuses on understanding behavior by discussing the helping relationship, growth and development, basic needs, and coping mechanisms. In Unit II the emphasis is on planning care for the individual client through a discussion of the details of a plan of care with an index of specific behaviors, goals, and approaches. This foundation for planning care is carried over into Unit III, in which specific patterns of behavior with sample plans of care are presented. It is in Units II and III that the above listed areas of concern are addressed. The sample plans of care provide a format for applying the theory of planning care to working with specific clients. The process of planning care then becomes more meaningful and challenging. Following an initial discussion of communication skills in Unit IV, there is a discussion of the various interventions that a health provider can use, individually or in a group setting, with some guidelines on stress management for the health provider. Unit V presents interventions for meeting specific needs of clients, and in Unit VI there are evaluation exercises that relate to the material that is covered in the book. These exercises can be used as pre- and post-assignments.

There is an increased emphasis today on education for all health providers, since it is recognized as an essential ingredient leading to effective performance. However, in all of the educational endeavors there is always a time element. Courses are being shortened. Time away from client care is carefully measured. It is our belief and the belief of those whom we have taught, both in the educational setting and in the work setting, that the simpler, more practical, and more realistic the material is, the quicker the health provider can see how it can be used in the clinical setting. We have tried to keep this in mind throughout the book.

BARBARA B. BAUER

SIGNE S. HILL

The following poem capsulizes the authors' beliefs regarding the essentials of mental health care.

Love begins when Acceptance is present.
Appreciation is an award shown by Praise.
Recognition is given when Goals are met.
Faith in oneself and others starts with Security.
Confidence grows when Encouragement smiles.
Patience thrives where Tolerance exists.
Forgiveness is a Privilege extended to all but enjoyed by few.
Truth is ever present where Honesty lives.
Justice has a way of finding its foundation of Fairness.
Education is a way of overcoming Ignorance.
Moderation is the safety valve of Indulgence.
Discipline is a series of sound investments in Character.
Kindliness is a priceless Commodity found in abundance
   among all peoples.
Friendliness is a boundless Freedom offered by the world in
   which we live.

AUTHOR UNKNOWN

ACKNOWLEDGMENTS

Numerous people participated in some way in the development of this book. We especially wish to thank the following:

—*Elizabeth Johnson*, a colleague who always kept her eyes open for a sales representative that might be interested in the book.

—*Dean Manke*, the area sales representative for W. B. Saunders Company who became excited by the purpose and proposed content of this book.

—*Ilze Rader*, our editor who has in turn been supportive, enthusiastic, persistent and yet eternally patient with us throughout the project.

—Our *reviewers* who provided valuable feedback and encouragement.

We also wish to acknowledge the following:

—*Amy Bauer Kaczynski*, who supplied the detailed original art work found in Chapters 2, 13, and 14 and helped enhance understanding of the material.

—*Paula Lamberg*, Behavior Analyst, who wrote Chapter 14 and made Grandma's Rule come alive.

—*Michael Hill*, Vocational Development Coordinator, who wrote the practical section on work therapy in Chapter 15.

—*Paul Schanen*, Registered Pharmacist, who contributed down-to-earth information for writing the section on psychopharmacology in Chapter 13.

—*Terri Timmers*, Registered Dietitian, who offered valuable insights that helped make the section on nutrition in Chapter 17 specific to the nutritional needs of clients with psychiatric problems.

—*Bonnie Kaminski*, LPN, for her creative use of the problem-solving steps in dealing with anxiety during her psychiatric rotation.

—*Carol J. Janus*, who staged and photographed the pictures in Chapter 18.

—*Marla Hill*, who helped to subdue the assaultive client seen in those photographs.

—*Robert G. Owens*, a clinical psychologist, who traveled many miles advocating for the mentally ill and imparting his caring techniques so that staff might have a better understanding of their clients' world.

—*Colleagues, students, clients,* and *staff,* whose needs provided the impetus to write this book.

Finally, we acknowledge that this project was indeed a family affair. Husband *George Bauer* located materials for us and untiringly edited what we wrote. Husband *Frank Hill* provided the original motif for the cover and unit pages and the wood for heating the cabin hideaway to which we disappeared to write. Our *children* (a total of seven) contributed directly as noted and indirectly by keeping us grounded in reality.

One final note: we acknowledge a friendship and professional relationship—ours—that has stood the test of working closely together and continually evaluating each other's work.

CONTENTS

UNIT III
SPECIFIC PATTERNS OF BEHAVIOR WITH SAMPLE PLANS OF CARE

UNIT IV
HEALTH PROVIDERS AND INTERVENTIONS

UNIT V
INTERVENTIONS TO MEET SPECIFIC NEEDS

UNIT VI
EVALUATION EXERCISES

UNIT I

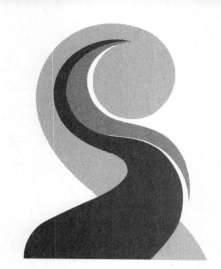

UNDERSTANDING
BEHAVIOR

PERSPECTIVES IN MENTAL HEALTH CARE

LEARNING OBJECTIVES—Upon completing this chapter, the reader will be able to:

1. Identify three treatment approaches for mentally ill persons, which reflect the values of the time.

2. Name five people who were significant to the mental health movement.

3. Identify the federal legislation that led to improvement in the care of the mentally ill.

4. Name two reports that contributed to increased public awareness of mental health problems.

5. Define *caring*.

6. Explain the significance of caring in working with the emotionally disturbed.

7. Describe five aspects of caring.

HISTORY OF THE MENTAL HEALTH MOVEMENT

The material covered in this history of the mental health movement focuses on areas that continue to be significant in the care of the mentally ill today. Such care, like other things in life, reflects the predominant values of the time (Angrist, 1963:20).

During the age of primitive man, all things, good and evil, were believed to have been caused by spirits. Incantations, spells, and charms were used to prevent or cure disease. The sorcerer was employed to cast out demons that were believed to cause all illness.

Four centuries before Christ, Hippocrates discarded the old theories and denied that mental disease was sacred. He felt that mental disorders, like other diseases, had natural causes and required treatment. During the third century B.C., Egyptian temples were the sites of purification treatment, plus various amusements and pleasurable activities, for the mentally ill. With the advent of Christianity, the Church began to provide care for the mentally ill and other patients in its monasteries. During the dark ages, little improvement is noted in caring for the mentally ill. At Gheel, Belgium, a system of colony care for the mentally ill was instituted. According to folklore and legend, an Irish princess, Dymphna, was slain in the area of Gheel in A.D. 600 by her insane, widowed father, the King, after she refused his request to marry him. Many people flocked to Dymphna's tomb in the hope that she might intercede on behalf of the ill. Miraculous cures were reported and as the Dymphna legend spread, Gheel became increasingly renowned as a center for the treatment of the mentally ill (Aring, 1974:849). As more and more people came to the village, they began to take housing with the townsfolk. Thus, the people of Gheel became accustomed to the mentally ill. Since the thirteenth century, the Colony of Gheel has been a haven for those with mental illness and has served as a model for community care in the United States.

The Renaissance and the Reformation brought new changes in the care of the mentally ill. Lunacy legislation appeared in England during the reign of King Edward II when a law was enacted that directed the property of lunatics to be vested in the crown. Founded in 1247, The Hospital of St. Mary of Bethlehem in London was one of the first places to provide care for the treatment of the mentally ill. (The hospital's name was later shortened to "Bedlam," a term which then entered the language in its present sense.)

In 1792, in Paris, Phillipe Pinel, in less than a week, liberated more than 50 patients who had been in chains for 30 years. He believed that these patients were unmanageable only because they had been robbed of their freedom, and the results proved that he was right. He provided workshops with light and air instead of the darkness and stench of the dungeons. William Tuke founded the York Retreat in England, an asylum for sick Quakers; and Dr. John Conolly, also of England, became an enthusiastic advocate of nonrestraint. In 1856, Dr. Conolly published a book, *The Treatment of the Insane Without Mechanical Restraint*, which established a new principle in hospital management. He wrote, "Restraints and neglect may be considered as synonymous; for restraints are merely a general substitute for the thousand attentions required by troublesome patients" (Conolly, 1973:323). After five years as superintendent of an asylum in England, during which time no mechanical restraint was used, he wrote, "there is no asylum in the world in which all mechanical restraints may not be abolished, not only with perfect safety, but with incalculable advantage" (Conolly, 1973:261).

In America, prior to the middle of the eighteenth century, many mentally ill individuals were confined to poorhouses and jails, where they were treated as paupers and common criminals. The first American hospital to care for mental patients along with other patients was the Pennsylvania Hospital in Philadelphia, established in 1752. The first public institution designed solely for the care of the mentally ill in the United States was opened at Williamsburg, Virginia, in 1773. Dr. Benjamin Rush was the first American physician to make a serious study of mental disorders and is considered the father of American Psychiatry. Along with Pinel of France and Tuke of England, he was influential in spreading the doctrine of moral treatment, which advocated treating the mentally ill with kindness and humanitarianism.

In spite of the reform movements for separate institutions and moral treatment, the facilities for the care of the mentally ill remained overcrowded and inadequate. In the middle of the nineteenth century, Dorothea Lynde Dix, a retired school teacher, agreed to teach Sunday School classes to women inmates. She was shocked at the filth, the apparent neglect and brutality, and the number of insane locked in cells. She aroused public opinion regarding the treatment of mental patients and campaigned for more and larger institutions for their care.

A number of people made significant contributions to psychiatry around the beginning of the twentieth century. Emil Kraepelin described mental illnesses and gave them names. He is sometimes referred to as the great descriptive psychiatrist. Sigmund Freud, founder of psychoanalysis, introduced the idea that unconscious motivation is important in causing mental illness.

A significant figure in the mental health movement was Clifford W. Beers, a graduate of Yale University, who spent three years as a patient in mental hospitals. Following his recovery, he was determined to do something about the conditions that existed in these hospitals. He accomplished this by writing an account of his experiences entitled *A Mind That Found Itself*. His exposé of mental institutions contributed directly to the organization of the mental hygiene movement. On May 6, 1909, Beers founded the Connecticut Society for Mental Hygiene. The chief purpose of the society was "to work for the conservation of mental health; to help prevent nervous and mental disorders and mental defects; to help raise the standards of care for those suffering from any of these disorders or defects; to secure and disseminate reliable information on these subjects; to cooperate with federal, state, and local agencies or officials and with public and private agencies whose work is in any way related to that of a society for mental hygiene" (Beers, 1948:304). The following year the National Committee for Mental Hygiene was organized. In 1950, it merged with the National Mental Health Foundation and the Psychiatric Foundation to form the National Association for Mental Health, Inc. The symbol of the Mental Health Association is the Mental Health Bell, which was cast from shackles and chains that once restrained people in mental hospitals. The 300 pound bell, housed in Arlington, Virginia, bears the inscription, CAST FROM THE SHACKLES WHICH BOUND THEM, THIS BELL SHALL RING OUT HOPE FOR THE MENTALLY ILL AND VICTORY OVER MENTAL ILLNESS.

At the beginning of the twentieth century, the mentally ill were usually cared for and treated in large state-run institutions. These institutions were often located outside the city, with the explanation that the patients needed the fresh country air. Frequently, however, it was the fear and stigma associated with mental illness that dictated the location of the institutions. Descriptive psychiatry provided the knowledge base for treatment. Symptoms of mental disorders were learned, and patients exhibiting those symptoms were slotted into the various diagnostic categories. The treatments given were classified as physical or medical therapies. These included insulin coma therapy, introduced by Sakel of Vienna in 1933; electroshock therapy for the artificial production of convulsive seizures, initiated by Cerletti and Bini of Italy in 1938; and prefrontal lobotomy, begun by Moniz and Lima of Portugal in 1936. Hydrotherapy continued to be used as it had been in ancient times to relax the body.

World War II brought about public and professional awareness of the effects of psychological stress and the widespread need for the rehabilitation of veterans. The public also recognized that mental illness was costing the taxpayers millions of dollars each year and that facilities for the care of these people were inadequate. These factors led to the passage of The National Mental Health Act in 1946. Its purpose was to provide federal aid for research, training, and community service. In 1948, the National Institute of Mental Health, located at the Clinical Center of the National Institutes of Health in Bethesda, Maryland, was created.

During the 1950s, psychotherapeutic drugs were introduced as a treatment for the mentally ill. They were not a "cure" for mental illness, but the drugs made the patient more amenable to other forms of psychotherapy. As a result of medication, patients began to move out of the large institutions. In 1961, the Joint Commission on Mental Illness and Health published a report entitled *Action for Mental Health*. The report placed strong emphasis on community-based services by calling for a reduction in the size of large state hospitals and the development of mental health services in local communities (Joint Commission, 1961:268). The Mental Retardation Facilities and Community Mental Health Centers Construction Act of 1963 provided funds for establishing a network of publicly funded community mental health centers throughout the country.

Thus, a movement called *deinstitutionalization* began. Large numbers of mental patients were moved out of state hospitals into the community. Many found themselves in worse conditions than in the institution, since the communities were not prepared to receive them. Chronically ill patients who needed rehospitalization would go to nursing homes. Nursing homes have been called "the new mental hospitals of America" (Pfeiffer, 1983:17). In 1977, the "President's Commission on Mental Health" was established to review the mental health needs of the nation and to make recommendations as to how those needs might best be met. Its report in 1978 focused on the following areas:

—Development of networks of high-quality mental health services at the local level, coordinating mental health services with other human services.

—Adequate financing of mental health services with public and private funds.

—Appropriately trained personnel.

—Services for populations with special needs.

—National priority to meet needs of people with chronic mental illness.

—An increased base of knowledge about the nature and treatment of mental disabilities.

—Protection of human rights and the guaranteeing of freedom of choice.

—Prevention of mental diseases.

In 1941, Gregory Zilboorg, in *A History of Medical Psychology*, wrote that "The history of psychiatry is essentially the history of humanism. Every time humanism has diminished or degenerated into mere philanthropic sentimentality, psychiatry has entered a new ebb. Everytime the spirit of humanism has arisen, a new contribution to psychiatry has been made" (Zilboorg, 1941:524–525). So in this age of humanism, the health provider is challenged to provide high-quality care for the emotionally distraught in the least restrictive environment, using the resources provided by their caregivers in their natural environment. High-quality care is related to the type of helping relationship that exists between the health provider and the client. The most effective helping relationship revolves around various aspects of caring.

The Helping Relationship—Aspects of Caring

Caring is a word used freely in the health field. It is part of the Salvation Army's slogan, "Caring Is Sharing," and has been used on buttons for National Nursing Home Week to express themes such as, "Care With Dignity" and "We Care." Books about health use "Caring" as part of the title, as in Leininger's (1981) *Caring: An Essential Human Need* and Mayeroff's (1971) *On Caring*. All of these references convey that caring is a dynamic process, an essential part of living. *Caring is the essence of the helping relationship,* and the helping relationship is the basic tool in working with clients who are emotionally disturbed.

Figure 1–1 depicts some of the aspects of caring that are meaningful in working with those who are emotionally disturbed. Since the most important tool used in working with an emotionally disturbed individual is one's self, one's personality, having a *knowledge* of one's self—one's needs, strengths, and limitations—is vital. Such knowledge prevents the health provider from imposing his value system upon the client or leading the client in the direction that the health provider desires rather than allowing the client's growth to be the guide. Having gained this knowledge of one's self, it is then important to understand the client's needs, strengths, and limitations; how to respond properly to them; and what would be helpful to the client's *growth* (Mayeroff, 1971:13).

These basic understandings prepare the health provider for this *involvement* in and *commitment* to the treatment of clients in psychiatric and nursing home settings. Working with the mentally ill is a person-to-person treatment in which the health provider uses his or her problem-solving skills to assist the client in exploring alternatives for dealing with his situation. One might say, "Look, you have five ways of dealing with this problem. This is the one you took. It didn't work out for you; it's not in your own best interest. So why not examine these other four?" This is the way the health provider becomes involved in the client's growth process and makes a commitment to caring—a commitment to get involved and not allow the client to wallow in his confusion; to say "Look, I care enough about you to interrupt your crazy behavior and help you behave in a more realistic and human way." This extension of oneself into the unknown without being certain of the outcome is *risky*. "But risk must be taken, because the greatest hazard in life is to risk *nothing*. The person who risks nothing does nothing, has nothing, and is nothing. He may avoid suffering and sorrow, but he simply cannot learn, feel, change, grow, live, or love. . . . Only the person who risks is free" (Buscaglia, 1982:264).

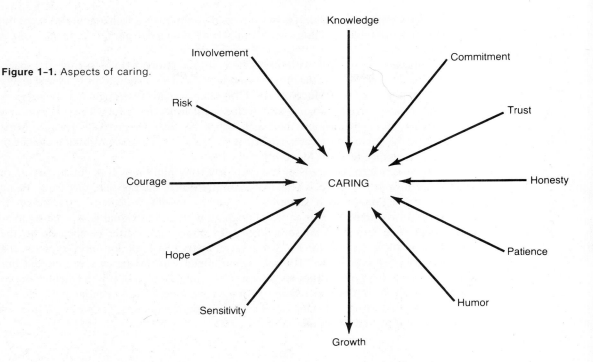

Figure 1–1. Aspects of caring.

In order to take a risk, one must have *trust* in oneself—confidence in one's ability to make decisions. If the health provider is continually preoccupied with whether his judgment was correct or not, he becomes indifferent to the client's needs. Once self-trust is established, one can begin to trust others, a step that involves letting go and allowing the individual to grow in his own way (Mayeroff, 1971:20–21).

It takes *courage* to trust the other person to grow, to allow that person to make mistakes and learn from them, and to venture into the unknown where all sorts of risk exist. The direction the health provider must take is sometimes unclear, but the knowledge of oneself, one's past experience, provides guidelines for the present situation. In using the knowledge about one's past experience, the health provider must always keep in mind that although the client's problems may sound similar to one the health provider has experienced, the client's problem belongs to him. Consequently, the solution that may have been right for the health provider may not be right for the client. The health provider's role is to guide the client through the problem-solving process at his level of functioning.

"*Honesty* is present in caring as something positive, and not as a matter of *not* doing something, not telling lies or not deliberately deceiving others" (Mayeroff, 1971:18). This aspect of caring is very significant in working with the mentally ill. Since the interpersonal relationship is the therapeutic tool that the health provider uses to facilitate growth in the client, this interaction must "ring true." In other words, the health provider's feelings and actions must coincide. If the health provider tells a client, "I really care about you," simply because he feels he should say it and not because he actually does care, the provider has been emotionally dishonest. Consequently, the client will not grow through his interaction with the health provider.

Hope is an important aspect in caring for the mentally ill because of the long term nature of the illness. It is hoped that the client will grow through the health provider's caring. Hope denotes activity and not passivity; it's "an expression of a present alive with possibilities" (Mayeroff, 1971:26). These possibilities consist of very small, realistic, measurable, and attainable goals; maybe it is just to get the client to look the health provider in the eye for a second. It is this tiny goal that triggers another goal and keeps the fire going. It is like building a house; each small brick is added to another until the house is completed.

It takes *patience* to work with the mentally ill, and patience involves time and space. Being patient means allowing the other person to grow in his own time and way and giving him room to think and feel. Mayeroff (1971:18) refers to it as "the patient man [who] gives the other room to live." Patience also includes tolerance for another's confusion and floundering and the realization that such behaviors also characterize growth. Most importantly, the person who cares is patient with himself. He gives himself a chance to learn—and a chance to care (Mayeroff, 1971:18).

Being *sensitive* to the needs of the client is letting him know that you are trying to understand how he feels. Such sensitivity communicates the message of caring. Being sensitive to the humor in a situation, yet having insight enough to understand its seriousness, also communicates caring. Laughing with an individual is not the same as laughing at him; laughter can sometimes help one gain a better perspective on the presenting problem. *Humor* can be used to facilitate trust in a relationship and establish a bond between the individuals. Humor "when joined with loving care can extend our humanity in reaching out to another person" (Osterlund, 1983:47). It is in reaching out to another that the health provider shares with the client one of life's essential ingredients— caring. "Through caring and being cared for man experiences himself as part of nature; we are closest to a person or an idea when we help it grow" (Mayeroff, 1971:87).

REFERENCES

Angrist, S.S., 1963. The mental hospital: Its history and destiny. Perspect Psychiatr Care, Vol. I, No. 6, pp. 20–26.

Aring, C.D., 1974. Gheel revisited. JAMA, Vol. 239, No. 7, Nov. 11, p. 849.

Beers, C.W., 1948. A Mind That Found Itself. 7th ed. New York, Doubleday and Company, Inc.

Buscaglia, L., 1982. Living, Loving, Learning. New York, Ballantine Books.

Conolly, J., 1856. Treatment of the Insane Without Mechanical Restraints. London: Smith, Elder and Company. Reprinted by photolithography in 1973 by Dawsons of Pall Mall, London, England.

Joint Commission on Mental Illness and Health, 1961. Action for Mental Health. New York, John Wiley and Sons, Inc.

Leininger, M., 1981. Caring: An Essential Human Need. Thorofare, N.J., Charles B. Slack, Inc.

May, R., 1969. Love and Will. New York, W.W. Norton and Company, Inc.

Mayeroff, M., 1971. On Caring. New York, Harper and Row Publishers.

Osterlund, H., 1983. Humor: A serious approach to patient care. Nursing 83, December, pp. 46–47.

Paulen, A., 1982. Commit yourself to caring. J Pract Nursing, January, pp. 26–27.

Pfeiffer, E., 1983. Assessments: The long term care issue of the '80s. Coordinator, July, p. 17.

The President's Commission on Mental Health, 1978. Report. Washington, D.C., U.S. Government Printing Office.

Slavinsky, A., 1984. Psychiatric nursing in the year 2000: From a nonsystem of care to a caring system. Image: J Nurs Scholarship, Winter, pp. 17–20.

Warner, S.L., 1984. Humor and self-disclosure within the milieu. J Psychosocial Nurs Ment Health Serv, April, pp. 17–21.

Zilboorg, G., 1941. A History of Medical Psychology. New York, W.W. Norton and Company, Inc.

RELATIONSHIP OF GROWTH AND DEVELOPMENT TO BEHAVIOR

LEARNING OBJECTIVES—Upon completing this chapter, the reader will be able to:

1. Name two persons who have contributed major theories of personality development.

2. Explain the relationship of needs to behavior.

3. Describe two ways of categorizing needs.

4. Explain what is meant by *id, ego,* and *superego.*

5. Identify the developmental tasks for each of Erikson's eight stages.

6. Discuss briefly each of the five stages of development according to Freud.

7. Describe five levels of needs based on Maslow's Theory of Needs.

8. Give one example for each of the 16 coping/mental mechanisms illustrated.

9. Utilize the problem-solving process in a familiar anxiety-provoking situation.

THEORIES RELATED TO THE LIFE CYCLE

It is through an understanding of human development that the health provider can distinguish between the client's chronological level and actual functioning level and, therefore, develop more realistic care plans. Although only Freud's and Erikson's theories are discussed at length in this book, it is worth noting that other theorists contributed a great deal of knowledge about personality development. For example, Harry Stack Sullivan emphasized the importance of self-esteem and believed that many mental disorders result from anxiety due to inadequate communication. Jean Piaget's contribution was a cognitive theory. Most of his research concerned how children learn and how they use what they learn in the adult world. B.F. Skinner is the person associated with behaviorism in the United States. His theory of operant conditioning implies that behavior is predictable but is also influenced by experience, interest and ability. Wolpe's behavior therapy uses the knowledge gained from the behavior theorists to change behavior through positive reinforcement. The humanistic theories of Carl Rogers and Abraham Maslow focus on the whole person, including the qualities that make people distinctive and how these qualities develop. Humanistic theory is a very optimistic view of man's nature and capabilities. Existentialistic theory is similar to humanistic theory but is less optimistic with regard to man. Rollo May emphasizes the person's individuality and identifies the significance in recognizing a higher order of being (Lancaster, 1983:41).

However, it was the work of Sigmund Freud that set into motion the study of human development, motivation, and thought. Since that time, his theories have been modified and have stimulated the development of new theories.

Originally, Freud's work, most of which was with adults, was intended to describe how individuals developed neurosis (minor mental illness). Later, his work became a general theory about human personality development. According to Freud, human personality has three parts: the *id*, the *ego*, and the *superego*.

He identified id as the part from which arise a person's primitive urges and instincts, such as sexual desires and aggression. Although unconscious, the id may have observable effects on a person's thinking, feeling, and behavior. Freud's theory stressed the *unconscious* nature of motivation and the powerful effect of the hidden sources of human behavior. Dreams, for example, can offer clues to unconscious motivation. The id, being unconscious, intrudes into our dreams and becomes an important source of revealing an individual's fundamental motives.

The ego, on the other hand, is conscious and operates on the reality principle: Postpone satisfaction to attain more important long-term goals. The ego provides some controls over the id, which wants to satisfy its every whim (pleasure principle) and would destroy the person in its continual demands to satisfy its urges. Consequently, impulse control and the guiding of behavior toward long-term goals is the ego's function.

The superego is sometimes thought of as the conscience. It is actually more than that. It is the place where the ego finds the rules it uses to control the id. It is primarily unconscious, incorporating the values of human society, and acts as a censor for the id. According to Saxton and Haring (1975:13), "if these parts of personality could speak, the conversation would probably follow these lines:

> Id: "I want what I want when I want it."
> Superego: "You can't have it."
> Ego: "Why not wait to see what tomorrow brings?"

The id, ego, and superego are not fixed. Instead, they are dependent upon the individual human experience and the adjustment that is achieved as a result of the pulling and tugging between instinctive urges and society's demands.

Erik Erikson developed his psychosocial theory of personality development from studying children. "Erikson formulated a theory of growth and development that includes the influences of Freud (biological, instinctual drives, libido), the influences of Sullivan (a student of Freud's who focused on social experience with significant persons who mold identity), and also a rationale for the cultural influences which we recognize today as influencing the way an individual experiences himself as a living entity" (Robinson, 1972:59). Freud's and Erikson's theories share some things in common and have outstanding differences as well. For example, both theories are based on orderly development that occurs in stages. Erikson's eight stages encompass the complete cycle from birth through old age. Freud's five stages extend from infancy to puberty (Kreigh and Perko, 1983:113–118). Erikson placed more emphasis on the need to solve problems at each stage of personality development. Freud placed more emphasis on the sex drive as a cause for negative behavior. Erikson believed that social and environmental factors influence personality development. He also emphasized healthy aspects of personality rather than pathology, as Freud did. In general, Erikson viewed human development more optimistically (Lancaster, 1980:22).

Table 2–1 offers a comparative look at Freud's and Erikson's theories of personality development.

TABLE 2-1.   A Comparative Look at Freud's and Erikson's Theories of Personality Development

Age	Theorist	Stage or Task	Commendable Quality	Undesirable Behavior	Significant Others
0–2 years	*FREUD*—Stage 1 Expresses needs and satisfaction through mouth: sucking, noises, crying, breathing	Oral stage	Weaning	Oral habits later in life such as overeating, drinking, cigarette smoking, nail-biting, gum chewing	Mother or mothering person
0–1 year	*ERIKSON*—Stage 1 Expresses needs through crying. Dependent on others to meet needs quickly and gently.	Trust versus mistrust	Hope	Frustration Fear Despair	
2–3 years	*FREUD*—Stage 2 Toilet training. First experience with mastery. Considered first experience with creativity.	Anal stage	Toilet training Self-control Responsibility	Parsimony Compulsiveness Obstinacy Possessiveness	Mother and father
1–3 years	*ERIKSON*—Stage 2 Learns to "do it him-self" (i.e., eating, walking, toileting)	Autonomy versus self-doubt and shame	Willpower	Feels dirty or bad Reckless bravado Shamelessness	
3–5 years	*FREUD*—Stage 3 Interest in genital area. Begins to under-stand sexual dif-ferences.	Phallic	Satisfaction with self as a sexual being Positive control over self Identify with same parent	Guilt and dis-satisfaction with self as a sexual being	Mother and father Playmates
5–6 years	Time of conflict. Needs to resolve attraction to op-posite parent and identify with same parent.	Oedipal			
3–6 years	*ERIKSON*—Stage 3 Still self-centered Shows off Looks for approval	Initiative versus guilt	Purpose Develops con-science Accepts con-sequences of acts	Feels morally bad Difficulty with decisions	
6–10 years	*FREUD*—Stage 4 Moral teaching from parents Confused in un-familiar settings Needs direction, approval, praise Sexual interest dormant	Latency	Sense of moral responsibility (superego)	Confusion regarding expectations	Peers Other adults
6–12 years	*ERIKSON*—Stage 4 Seeks achievement Interacts with others Sometimes competes	Industry versus inferiority	Competence Completes activities that are begun	Feels mediocre Withdraws Acts out	
11–13 years	*FREUD*—Stage 5 Puberty Biologic changes and drives Time of confusion and turmoil	Genital	Control of biologic drives Education and economic goals Privacy important	Unresolved confusion and turmoil regard-ing biologic changes and drives	

Table continues on following page.

TABLE 2–1. A Comparative Look at Freud's and Erikson's Theories of Personality Development (Continued)

Age	Theorist	Stage or Task	Commendable Quality	Undesirable Behavior	Significant Others
11–13 years	FREUD—Stage 5 (continued) Education and economic goals important Drives take second place				
12–18 or 21 years	ERIKSON—Stage 5 Great physical and emotional changes Anxiety and mood swings typical	Identity versus role confusion	Fidelity Learns who he is and what he can and cannot do and knows what others think of him	Problems with sexual role Delinquent behaviors Delinquent in choosing a career or vocation Problems with interpersonal relationships	Peers Adult role models
21–35 or 40 years	ERIKSON—Stage 6 Establishes intimate personal relationships with friends Establishes intimate love relationship with one person	Intimacy versus isolation	Love Mature relationship with member of opposite sex Suitable marital partner Performs work and socializes in acceptable ways	Isolation from others: Unable to share feelings, thoughts, and needs on emotionally mature level	Spouse Children
35 or 40 to 65 years	ERIKSON—Stage 7 Marriage/family or fulfillment through career, religious vocation, etc. Children leave home Begins to be concerned about what will happen to future generations	Generativity versus stagnation	Care Involvement in helping activities Creative, caring, productive	Overly concerned with bodily changes and self Selfish Exploits others Parasitic existence	Community Other generations
65 years to death	ERIKSON—Stage 8 Satisfaction with one's achievements	Integrity versus despair	Wisdom Reviews life realistically Accepts past failures and future limitations Helps younger generation view life realistically Accepts death with dignity	Sees past as total failure Fears death	Self

HUMAN NEEDS AND BEHAVIOR

Freud's and Erikson's theories of personality development are only two of the many theories about the growth process that attempt to explain why people are as they are and how they develop as individuals. Basically, the theorists agree that development occurs in an orderly progression through specific stages, from conception through death. This orderly progression is a dynamic process for each individual, based on his uniqueness. This

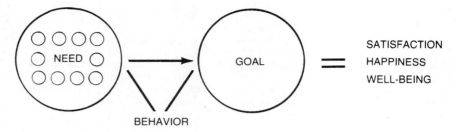

Figure 2-1. Results of goal achievement.

uniqueness is a combination of an individual's inherent potential, his past experiences, and the environment in which he lives. All of these factors create specific needs within an individual's life. It is how one deals with these needs that determines how effectively he moves through the life cycle. Therefore, a basic understanding of needs is essential in order to plan care for clients with psychiatric problems.

Needs are like holes in an individual's life, which, when filled, result in an increased feeling of well being. A goal is the point toward which one directs his efforts in order to fulfill his need. The activity that results from an individual's moving toward his goal to fulfill his need is one description of behavior.

Figure 2-1 shows that satisfaction, happiness, and well-being are experienced when the goal is achieved.

Figure 2-2 diagrams what happens when an obstacle is encountered along the pathway to the goal. Frustration and anxiety are experienced. These feelings are normal reactions to obstacles throughout the life cycle. As vague and uncomfortable as these feelings may be, they can be growth-producing if dealt with in a constructive, problem-solving way. If constructive ways are not used, the individual may experience distress and find destructive ways of coping with the discomfort. At this point the health provider must intervene and help the individual utilize the problem-solving process.

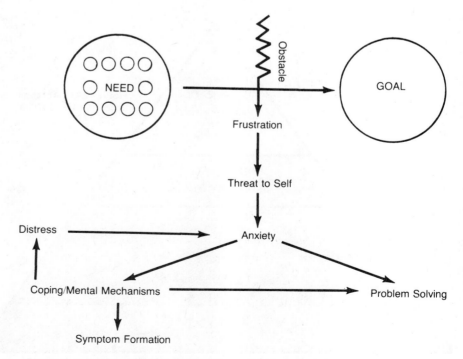

Figure 2-2. Results of interference with goal achievement.

EXAMPLE

The health provider is reassigned to another work area in which he does not feel competent. He is afraid to share this information with his supervisor for fear of receiving a poor evaluation. The health provider goes home with a headache (symptom formation). Unless the health provider risks confronting the supervisor and working through his problem, he will continue to have symptom formation using the mechanism of conversion.

Therefore, **all** behavior is **purposeful** and **meaningful**. Hence the observation of behavior is a source for assessing an individual's needs.

Needs can be categorized in many ways. One way is to consider them in relation to the physical, emotional, social, intellectual, and spiritual aspects of an individual's life.

Physical needs, sometimes referred to as biological needs, are closely related to body function and are necessary for survival. They include food, water, air, clothing, shelter, sex, exercise, and sensory and motor stimulation. At each stage of development, the individual finds new ways to satisfy his needs. In the infant, the mother provides food, warmth, and stimulation. As the child grows, he finds other ways to meet his basic physical needs based on his previous experiences. Emotional needs are "the need to love and be loved and the need to feel that we are worthwhile to ourselves and to others" (Glasser, 1965:9). It is through love that the individual receives approval and esteem; it is through feeling worthwhile that an individual gains respect and feels that he is a contributing member of society. Social needs evolve from the individual's cultural group. The most common social need is identification or belonging. During adolescence, belonging to a peer group is very important. Intellectual or learning needs begin at birth. Survival and security are related to the learning of specific tasks during the various stages of development. Spiritual needs are also related to the individual's cultural influences and can have a significant effect on his behavior.

Another way of viewing needs, known as the Hierarchy of Needs (Figure 2-3), was presented by psychologist Abraham Maslow. Maslow maintained that the most powerful,

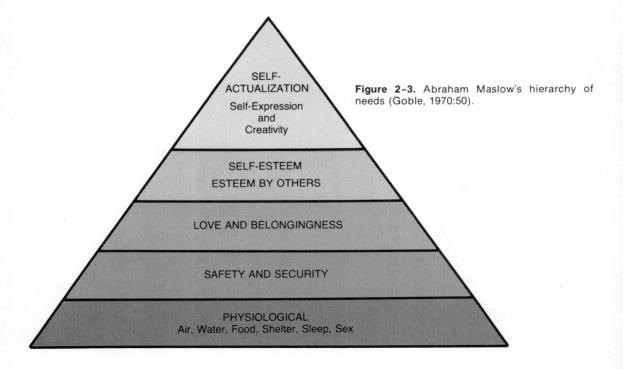

Figure 2-3. Abraham Maslow's hierarchy of needs (Goble, 1970:50).

basic needs are those of physical survival, such as food, water, shelter, sex, sleep, and air. After the needs at this level are reasonably satisfied, the individual then moves to the next level of safety and security, which includes the need for protection. Upon fulfillment of these needs, the individual is motivated to go on to the third level of belongingness and love. At this level the individual feels a need for belonging to a group, for acceptance, and for being able to give of one's self. The fourth level focuses on self-esteem and addresses the need for feelings of self-reliance, self-respect, confidence, and self-trust. According to Maslow, the first four levels cover basic needs. Remaining levels relate to Growth Needs, which center on self-actualization, the ultimate in need fulfillment (Goble, 1970:36–51).

The following anonymous poem graphically portrays the growth process and the impact that basic needs can have on behavior:

> After a while you learn
> the subtle difference
> between holding a hand
> and chaining a soul.
> And you learn
> that love doesn't mean leaning
> and company doesn't mean security.
> And you begin to learn
> that kisses aren't contracts
> and presents aren't promises.
> And you begin to accept your defeats
> with your head up and your eyes ahead
> with the grace of a woman or a man,
> not the grief of a child,
> and learn to build all your roads on today
> because tomorrow's ground is
> too uncertain for plans,
> and futures have a way of falling down
> in mid-flight.
> After a while you learn
> that even sunshine burns if you ask too much.
> So you plant your own garden
> and decorate your own soul
> instead of waiting for someone to bring you flowers.
> And you learn
> that you really can endure
> that you really are strong
> and you really do have worth.
> And you learn
> and you learn
> with every goodbye
> you learn. . . . . .
>
> AUTHOR UNKNOWN

COPING/MENTAL MECHANISMS

Coping/mental mechanisms (defense mechanisms) are unconscious ways of dealing with discomfort. Many of them develop early in childhood when the individual is placed in stressful situations that he cannot handle. In an effort to survive, the individual develops unconscious, automatic coping devices. Depending upon the degree to which they are used, they can have a healthy or unhealthy effect on the individual. These mechanisms continue to be active throughout a person's life, even when the original stress no longer exists. The following coping mechanisms will be briefly defined and illustrated:

Compensation	Projection
Conversion	Rationalization
Denial	Reaction formation
Displacement	Regression
Dissociation	Repression
Fantasy	Sublimation
Identification	Symbolization
Introjection	Undoing

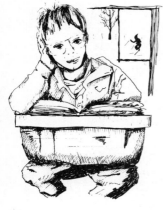

Compensation is covering for real or imagined inadequacy by developing or exaggerating a desirable trait. *Example:* An undersized boy develops his intellectual ability instead of participating in sports.

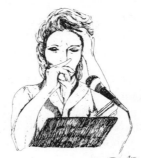

Conversion is the channeling of anxiety into physical symptoms. *Example:* Mrs. Smith develops a headache on the evening she is scheduled to present a paper at a convention and is unable to make her presentation.

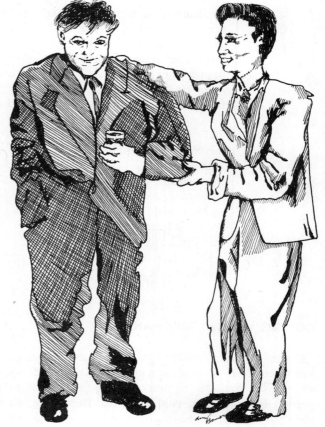

Denial is the rejection of things, events, or feelings as they actually are, thus eliminating the need for anxiety. *Example:* The alcoholic denies his alcoholism. "I am a social drinker and can stop anytime."

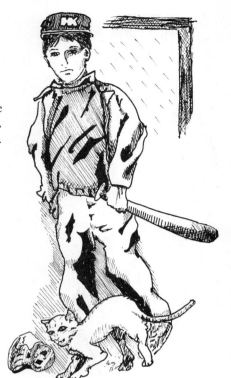

Displacement occurs when feelings toward an object are distorted and transferred to a less threatening object. *Example:* A boy, angry at the weather, which he cannot control, kicks his cat.

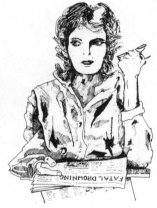

Dissociation occurs when painful ideas, situations, or feelings are separated from awareness. *Example:* Carol has forgotten details of the accident in which a loved one was killed.

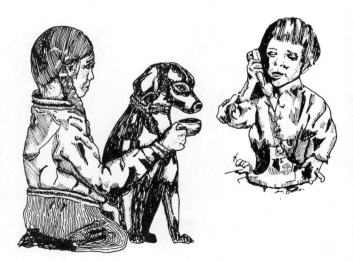

Fantasy is using the imagination to solve problems. On the conscious level, fantasy is used to reduce stress through relaxation. On the unconscious level, fantasy is used as a retreat from a threatening environment. *Example:* Children work through situations they will encounter in adult life by assuming parental roles and using their pets as children.

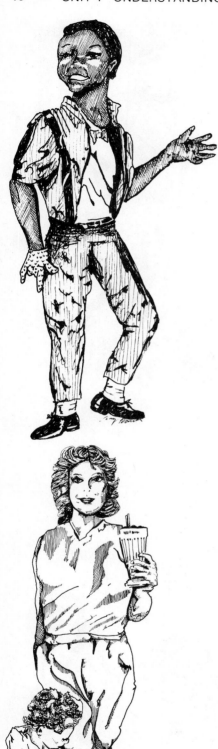

Identification occurs when an individual takes on the characteristics and values of someone he admires, recognizing that he is not that person. *Example:* Leon, age 15, dresses like his favorite singing star.

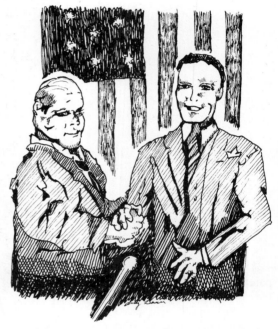

Introjection is the incorporating or internalizing of conflicting values, standards, persons, objects, or attitudes so that they are no longer an external threat. *Example:* A political candidate professes to represent every interest group so that none can attack his platform.

Projection is attributing to other people or objects motives and emotions that are unacceptable to oneself. *Example:* An overweight woman blames her two-year-old child for her condition saying that he makes her nervous.

Rationalization offers logical-sounding excuses that conceal the real reason for actions, thoughts, or feelings. *Example:* A young boy explains why he left for school without feeding the dog: "I did it because Johnny came over and told me we had to leave right away."

Reaction formation, sometimes viewed as an overcompensation, is a means of disguising from the self an unacceptable desire or drive by developing its exact opposite to an exaggerated degree. *Example:* The wife is angry at her husband for the attention he gives the dog but reacts by being overly sweet.

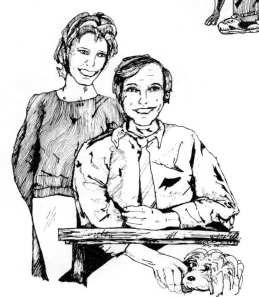

Regression is a retreat to an earlier, less stressful time of development. *Example:* An adult has a temper tantrum.

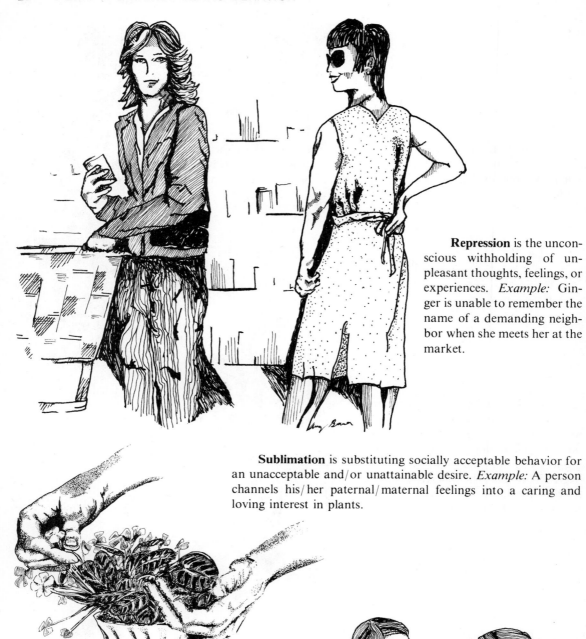

Repression is the unconscious withholding of unpleasant thoughts, feelings, or experiences. *Example:* Ginger is unable to remember the name of a demanding neighbor when she meets her at the market.

Sublimation is substituting socially acceptable behavior for an unacceptable and/or unattainable desire. *Example:* A person channels his/her paternal/maternal feelings into a caring and loving interest in plants.

Symbolization is the representation of an internal feeling, wish, attitude, or idea through an external object or quality (e.g., color). *Example:* A diamond ring and its presentation symbolize love and commitment.

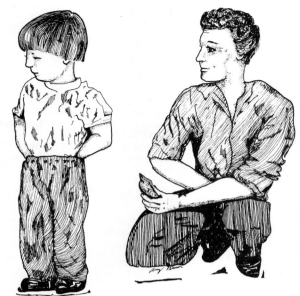

Undoing is an attempt to conceal negative action by other positive action. *Example:* A father offers his son an allowance after punishing him.

PROBLEM-SOLVING PROCESS

The problem-solving process is a conscious growth-producing method of dealing with stressful situations. By confronting the felt anxiety, the individual is able to move through the stressful situation. Steps in the problem-solving process include:

STEPS	EXAMPLE
1. Define the problem. What is actually causing the discomfort? Sometimes the problem is difficult to pinpoint.	A health provider has lost interest in going to work, is easily irritated, and over-reacts to clients' behaviors and requests.
2. Decide on a goal.	Regain interest in work.
3. Identify alternatives. (There is always more than one way to solve a problem.)	a. Quit his job. b. Ask for a transfer. c. Suggest to supervisor a change in assignment. d. Evaluate personal life cycle.
4. Choose an alternative.	Examine personal life cycle (ways of dealing with stress). a. Get involved in physical activities after work. —Return to swimming three times a week. —Rejoin volleyball league. b. Make a concerted effort not to think about work at home. c. Develop friendships outside of work setting.
5. Try out the alternatives.	Sign up for swimming at the YMCA. Join the volleyball league at church and tell self firmly, "When I'm at home I'll not think about work." Help the young people who moved in next door.
6. Evaluate the effectiveness.	Felt more relaxed after the exercise, slept well, felt refreshed upon awakening. Continued to have difficulty in not thinking about work at home. New neighbors seem interesting. Irritability at work is decreasing.
7. Repeat the process if the solution is not effective.	Solution to problem is helping. Need more time to evaluate.

REFERENCES

Broadribb, V., 1983. Introductory Pediatric Nursing. 3rd ed. Philadelphia, J.B. Lippincott Co.

Crawford, A., and Buchanan, B.B., 1974. Psychiatric Nursing, A Basic Manual. 4th ed. Philadelphia, F.A. Davis Co.

Erikson, E., 1963. Childhood and Society. New York, W.B. Norton and Co., Inc.

Glasser, W., 1965. Reality Therapy. New York, Harper and Row Publishers.

Goble, F., 1970. The Third Force: The Psychology of Abraham Maslow. New York, Grossman Publishers.

Lancaster, J., 1983. Adult Psychiatric Nursing. New York, Medical Examination Publishing Co., Inc.

Payne, D., and Clunn, P., 1977. Psychiatric Mental Health. 2nd ed. New York, Nursing Medical Examination Publishing Co., Inc.

Perko, J.E., and Kreigh, H., 1983. Psychiatric and Mental Health Nursing: A Commitment to Care and Concern. 2nd ed. Virginia, Reston Publishing Co., Inc.

Robinson L., 1972. Psychiatric Nursing as a Human Experience. 3rd ed. Philadelphia, W.B. Saunders Co., 1983.

Saxton, D., and Haring, P., 1975. Care of Patients with Emotional Problems. St. Louis, C.V. Mosby Co.

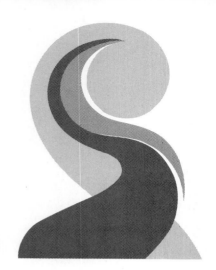

UNIT II

PLANNING CARE BASED ON STRENGTHS, NEEDS, PROBLEMS AND GOALS

CLASSIFICATION OF MENTAL DISORDERS AND PATTERNS OF BEHAVIOR

LEARNING OBJECTIVES—Upon completing this chapter, the reader will be able to:

1. Describe briefly each of the eight most commonly occurring mental disorders.

2. Identify the predominant behavior pattern of each *DSM-III* classification.

Emphasis in this book is on assisting the health provider to identify client behavior and to intervene in a helpful way. Clients may have more than one disturbed pattern of behavior during the course of an illness. The health provider will be able to respond to the client's needs more fully by learning to identify the pattern or patterns of behavior rather than relying solely on the diagnosis. However, the significance of classifying mental disorders cannot be overlooked. A medical diagnosis provides a way of sharing information that has specific meaning to all health providers. It is also important in determining treatment and prognosis, in maintaining statistics, and in collecting third-party payments.

The third edition of the *Diagnostic and Statistical Manual of Mental Disorders (DSM-III)*, published in 1980 by the American Psychiatric Association, lists a total of 16 major diagnostic classes and 187 specific diagnostic categories. A brief description of eight major mental disorders according to *DSM-III* follows.

1. ORGANIC MENTAL DISORDERS

Changes in organic functioning, whether due to injury or disease, substance use, the aging process, or medication therapy, can produce either temporary or permanent brain damage. Signs and symptoms may vary greatly according to the cause of the disorder and the extent of damage. Initial symptoms may include:

a. Changes in both recent and past memory, with past memory remaining intact for a longer period of time
b. Disorientation to time, place, and person
c. Various marked changes in intellectual functioning, including:
   1. Changes in affect (mood or emotion)
   2. Disorganization of thought
   3. Inappropriate behavior.

These latter symptoms are thought to represent an exaggeration of the individual's basic personality.

Delirium and dementia are two of the most common and important organic brain dysfunctions. *Delirium* is characterized by clouding of consciousness. For example, the client has difficulty focusing attention and is easily distracted. The onset is usually rapid, and additional symptoms, such as anxiety, incoherent speech, hallucinations, and increased or decreased psychomotor activity, may occur. The episode is usually brief, and recovery is complete if the underlying cause, such as substance intoxication, is treatable or self-limited. In the past, the term *dementia* meant a progressive, irreversible organic brain syndrome. The term as used in *DSM-III* is defined as "progressive, static or remitting" (APA, 1980:108). Memory impairment begins with short-term memory loss and may go on to include long-term memory loss, depending on the nature of the dementia. "*Primary Degenerative Dementia* of the Alzheimer type is the most common Dementia" (APA, 1980:110). Behavioral disorders may accompany impairment in thinking, judgment, and intellect in this progressive condition. The most common onset is after age 65; in most cases the brain atrophies. If the disorder occurs before age 65, it is called presenile onset. No treatment for dementia is available at this time, and most individuals will eventually need assistance in meeting their basic daily needs.

2. SUBSTANCE USE DISORDERS

Substance abuse is pathological use of a substance, even though the individual is aware of the harm to himself. Chemical substances that alter mood or depress or stimulate the central nervous system and those that are abused and/or cause dependence are included in this category. Repeated use of such substances results in problems with interpersonal relationships, job functioning, poor judgment and impulse control, changes in behavior, and, for some, involvement in criminal activity. The abusing individual deteriorates in both physical and psychological functioning. *Substance dependence* means that the user experiences physiological dependence, evidenced by tolerance or withdrawal. *Tolerance* indicates that increasing amounts of the drug are needed to achieve the desired effect. For example, an individual dependent on alcohol will report that the amount of alcohol he consumes before getting drunk has increased greatly over a period of time. *Withdrawal* refers to the syndrome (a set of symptoms specific to the substance) experienced by the user when the amount of drug is decreased or discontinued. The course of withdrawal also varies, depending on the drug. For example, withdrawal from heroin is uncomfortable, but death rarely occurs unless the individual has a severe physical condition such as heart disease. On the other hand, withdrawal from alcohol and barbiturates, both central nervous system depressants, could result in death in the absence of adequate medical supervision.

3. SCHIZOPHRENIC DISORDERS

Schizophrenic disorders, usually referred to as *schizophrenia,* actually comprise a large group of disorders, probably of different origins, that constitute a major health problem. A specific characteristic of these illnesses is deterioration from a previous level of functioning. Family or friends may note that the individual is "not the same." The client also experiences psychosis (being out of touch with reality) during the active phase of the illness. Some symptoms include delusions (false beliefs not supported by logic); hallucinations (hearing voices is most common); a blunted, flat, or inappropriate affect (mood or emotion not fitting to the situation); difficulty in making decisions that can result in not being able to function and care for oneself; and a deterioration in social relationships. Onset is during adolescence or early childhood. A residual phase follows the active phase, meaning that the person is left with an impairment in some activities of daily living, such as work, interpersonal relationships, or self-care. In the revised classification system, an individual cannot be classified as having schizophrenia unless he has had the symptomatology characteristic of this disorder for at least six months. Consequently schizophrenia is viewed as a chronic condition.

Individuals who are psychotic and who experience schizophrenia-like symptoms for more than two weeks and less than six months are now diagnosed as having a *schizophreniform disorder*. These individuals, whose symptoms are of short duration, are also more likely to return to their previous level of functioning. An acute onset of psychotic symptoms lasting at least a few hours but less than two weeks, with the cause identified, is now termed *brief reactive psychosis*. Both of these disorders are listed under "Psychotic Disorders not Elsewhere Classified" in the *DSM-III*.

Table 3–1 identifies the types of schizophrenic disorders and the diagnostic criteria according to *DSM-III*.

4. PARANOID DISORDERS

Paranoid disorders develop insidiously, generally in middle or late adult life, and are chronic conditions. The exception is the *acute paranoid disorder*, which develops suddenly and rarely becomes chronic. A firmly fixed (unshakable) delusion of persecution or jealousy develops, and the individual acts on that delusion by trying to "right wrongs" through complaints, letter writing, or legal action. The additional components of resentment and anger may lead the person to act violently. His thinking is clear and orderly in other areas, and he usually does not see himself as needing treatment. His introduction to the mental health system will most often be through family, a business associate, or the law. The *shared paranoid disorder* (folie à deux) develops as a result of a close relationship

TABLE 3–1. Schizophrenic Disorders and Diagnostic Criteria

TYPES OF SCHIZOPHRENIC DISORDER	DIAGNOSTIC CRITERIA ACCORDING TO *DSM-III*
Schizophrenia— Disorganized type	Frequent incoherence Absence of systematized delusions Blunted, inappropriate, or silly affect
Schizophrenia— Catatonic type	Any of the following: Catatonic stupor Catatonic negativism Catatonic rigidity Catatonic excitement Catatonic posturing
Schizophrenia— Paranoid type	One or more of the following: Persecutory delusions Grandiose delusions Delusional jealousy Hallucinations with persecutory or grandiose content
Schizophrenia— Undifferentiated type	Delusions Hallucinations Incoherence Loosening of associations Grossly disorganized behavior
Schizophrenia— Residual type	History of at least one previous episode of schizophrenia with prominent psychotic symptoms Clinical nature without any predominant symptoms Continuing evidence of illness such as blunted or inappropriate affect, social withdrawal, eccentric behavior, illogical behavior, or loosening of associations

Data from Diagnostic and Statistical Manual of Mental Disorders. 3rd ed. Washington, D.C., *The American Psychiatric Association,* 1980, pp. 190–193.

with another person who already has an established paranoid psychosis. "When the partners in this 'folie à deux' are separated, the dependent one recovers quickly, the dominant one does not" (Payne and Clunn, 1977:94). The *acute paranoid disorder* is seen in people who have changed their living or work situation. Examples of this would be young people leaving home for the first time, immigrants, or prisoners of war.

5. AFFECTIVE DISORDERS

Affective disorders, meaning "mood disorders," are characterized by depressive or manic (elated) episodes or both. During *major depressive episodes,* all processes (thinking, feeling, and doing) are slowed down. Contemplating or attempting suicide is not unusual when going into or coming out of a depression. During *manic episodes,* all processes speed up. Some persons switch from one behavior to another during the same illness (*mixed*).

Table 3–2 compares characteristics of manic and depressive episodes according to *DSM-III.*

6. ANXIETY DISORDERS

Anxiety is a universal emotion and is a threat only when it overwhelms. *Anxiety disorders,* previously listed as neuroses, arise when the individual does not resolve his or her problems in a positive way. In order to cope with the overwhelming anxiety, the

TABLE 3–2. Characteristics of Manic and Depressive Episodes

MANIC EPISODE	DEPRESSIVE EPISODE
1. More active than usual—demonstrates social, sexual, physical, or work-related restlessness	1. Loss of energy, fatigability, or tiredness
2. More talkative than usual or feels pressured to keep talking	2. Psychomotor agitation or retardation
3. Flight of ideas or subjective experience that thoughts are racing	3. Complaints or evidence of diminished ability to think or concentrate, such as slowed thinking or indecisiveness
4. Inflated self-esteem	4. Feelings of self-reproach or excessive or inappropriate guilt (either may be delusional)
5. Decreased need for sleep	5. Sleep difficulty or sleeping too much
6. Distractibility (i.e., attention is too easily drawn to unimportant or irrelevant external stimuli)	6. Recurrent thoughts of death or suicide or any suicidal behavior, including thoughts of wishing to be dead
7. Excessive involvement in activities without recognizing the high potential for painful consequences (i.e., buying sprees, sexual indiscretions, foolish business investments, reckless driving)	7. Loss of interest or pleasure in usual activities, or decrease in sexual drive
	8. Poor appetite or weight loss or increased appetite or weight gain (change of one pound a week or ten pounds a year when not dieting)

Data from Diagnostic and Statistical Manual of Mental Disorders. 3rd ed. Washington, D.C., The American Psychiatric Association, 1980, pp. 208, 214.

individual may separate (dissociate) the anxiety from the rest of his personality. The resulting symptoms give clues (symbolism) to the underlying problem, of which he is not consciously aware.

Phobic disorders (or phobic neuroses) are recognized by a persistent exaggerated fear of a specific object, activity, or situation. The person avoids whatever is feared. In some cases, the fear may be severe enough to prevent him from engaging in and enjoying normal daily activities, even though he realizes that the fear is unreasonable. Symptoms of *anxiety states* (or anxiety neuroses) vary according to the particular type of disorder. For example, individuals with a *panic disorder* may have recurring panic (anxiety) attacks and experience intense terror, feelings of impending doom, dyspnea, palpitations, chest pain, smothering sensation, dizziness, tingling of hands and feet, sweating, and faintness. Because the symptoms resemble physical disease, the patient is often first seen by his personal physician or in an emergency room. *Obsessive-compulsive disorders* are another type of anxiety neurosis. The obsessions are repetitive, unacceptable ideas such as killing one's child, and the compulsions are repetitive acts performed in an exact pattern used to relieve the anxiety produced by the obsessive thoughts. An example of a common compulsion is handwashing. When the person attempts not to give in to the compulsion, the mounting tension is overwhelming and can be immediately relieved by giving in to the act. Any interference with the person's compulsion will only increase his anxiety. The individual is aware of the ridiculousness of the obsessions or compulsions but is unable to control them. Persons experiencing sleep disturbance, memory impairment, or loss of concentration following a psychologically stressful event (such as rape, war, torture, flood) may be suffering from *post-traumatic stress disorder.*

7. SOMATOFORM DISORDERS

An alternative way of dealing with unresolved anxiety is to "bind" the anxiety (i.e., fix it onto the body). Individuals with somatoform disorders exhibit physical symptoms without having an organic disease. The *somatization disorder* is a common, chronic disorder that begins early in life. Dramatic, vague complaints and a complicated medical history with symptoms severe enough to require medication are part of the pattern. Often the individual has been or is being treated by more than one doctor. In the *psychogenic pain disorder,* the individual again expresses unresolved emotional problems through physical symptoms. The pain permits him to avoid some undesirable activity and to get support from his environment that he can't get otherwise. In *hypochondriasis,* the person is preoccupied with the thought of having a serious disease.

8. PERSONALITY DISORDERS

Personality disorders are ingrained maladaptive ways of dealing with stress. They show up in adolescence or earlier and continue through most of adult life. For some reason, they become less obvious in middle and old age. Individuals with a *histrionic personality disorder* behave dramatically, as if "on stage." Their reactions are out of proportion to the situation at hand. They are demanding and inconsiderate, use manipulative suicide attempts or threats, and tend to be seductive.

Persons with a *compulsive personality disorder* are "stiff" in their interpersonal contacts; perfectionistic, which often keeps them from completing tasks; and insistent that others do things their way. The *passive-aggressive personality disorder* is characterized by the person's resistance to performing adequately both socially and occupationally. The method of resisting is indirect and can be expressed through procrastination, dawdling,

TABLE 3-3. *DSM III and Related Patterns of Behavior*

CLASSIFICATION OF DISORDERS—*DSM III*	PATTERNS OF PREDOMINANT BEHAVIOR DESCRIBED IN THIS BOOK
Disorders usually first evident in infancy, childhood and adolescence	*Behavior pattern related to mental retardation and emotional disturbances*
Mental retardation	A developmental disorder characterized by below-normal intellect and complicated by emotional problems
Attention deficit disorder	
Conduct disorder	
Anxiety disorders of childhood or adolescence	
Eating disorders	*Children with an emotionally disturbed pattern of behavior*
Stereotyped movement disorders	Characterized by behaviors beyond those accepted as age-related behaviors
Other disorders with physical manifestations	
Pervasive development disorders	
Specific development disorders	
Organic mental disorders—organic brain syndrome	*Behaviors related to organic changes in the brain*
Delirium	Characterized by changes in judgment, memory; confusion, disorientation due to organic brain damage
Dementia	
Intoxication	
Withdrawal	
Organic mental disorders	
Dementias arising in the senium or presenium	
Primary degenerative dementia	
Substance-induced organic mental disorders	
Substance use disorders	*Behavior pattern related to the use of alcohol/ drugs*
Substance abuse	Characterized by extremely undesirable behavioral changes due to use of substances that affect the central nervous system
Substance dependence	
Schizophrenic disorders	*Withdrawal pattern of behavior*
Disorganized	Characterized by replacing reality with a world of one's own
Catatonic	
Paranoid	*Behavior patterns of the young, chronically mentally ill*
Undifferentiated	Characterized by a combination of many behaviors that are often psychotic
Residual	
Paranoid disorders	*Overly suspicious pattern of behavior*
Paranoia	Characterized by a greater than normal lack of trust that interferes with interpersonal relationships and activities of daily living
Shared paranoid disorder	
Acute paranoid disorder	
Psychotic disorders not elsewhere classified	
Schizophreniform disorder	
Brief reactive psychosis	
Schizoaffective disorder	

stubbornness, intentional inefficiency, or forgetfulness. The person with an *antisocial personality disorder* is in continuous social or legal trouble and appears to profit little from parental or social punishment. He tends to spend more time in the prison system than in the hospital system. Characteristics of the *borderline personality disorder* are manifested by impulsive behavior, sudden mood changes, unstable interpersonal relationships, and unpredictable actions that could be self-damaging. Such individuals experience chronic feelings of emptiness or boredom. The *schizotypal personality disorder* is similar to that previously known as schizophrenia, simple type. Many of these individuals make a marginal adjustment in the community. Most individuals with personality disorders do not seek treatment or require hospitalization unless they have an additional disorder. The last three disorders are the exception. Individuals with these disorders do not adjust readily to the community because of their maladaptive behavior and, therefore, move in and out of the mental health system.

For the health provider's convenience, the *DSM-III* is presented in an abbreviated form with the predominant pattern identified opposite the appropriate classification (Table 3-3). A brief definition of the pattern of behavior is included. Additional information about the classification of disorders can be obtained directly from the *DSM-III* manual, listed in the references at the end of the chapter.

TABLE 3-3. *DSM III* **and Related Patterns of Behavior** *(continued)*

CLASSIFICATION OF DISORDERS—*DSM III*	PATTERNS OF PREDOMINANT BEHAVIOR DESCRIBED IN THIS BOOK

Affective disorders
  Major affective disorders
    Manic episode
    Major depressive episode
  Bipolar disorder:
    Mixed
    Manic
    Depressed
	Overactive pattern of behavior
	  Characterized by overt aggressive behavior
	  exhibited by intensified mood, verbaliza-
	  tion, and frantic activity
	Depressive pattern of behavior
	  Characterized by feelings of unworthiness,
	  self-deprecation, hopelessness, help-
	  lessness, and morbid sadness.
	  This may be exhibited by:
	  1. Retarded depressive behavior
	  2. Agitated depressive behavior
	Suicidal pattern of behavior
	  Characterized by any self-destructive
	  pattern of behavior

Anxiety disorders
  Phobic disorders (Phobic neuroses)
  Anxiety states (anxiety neuroses)
  Panic disorder
  Obsessive/compulsive disorder
  Post-traumatic stress disorder
	Anxious pattern of behavior
	  Characterized by free-floating anxiety; vague
	  feelings of impending doom accompanied
	  by physical symptoms, such as
	  diaphoresis, tachycardia, and
	  gastrointestinal symptoms

Somatoform disorders
  Somatization disorder
  Conversion disorder
  Psychogenic pain disorder
  Hypochondriasis
Dissociative disorder
  Psychogenic amnesia
  Multiple personality
Psychosexual disorders
  Gender identity disorders
  Paraphilias
  Psychosexual dysfunctions	

Personality disorders
  Schizotypal
  Histrionic
  Antisocial
  Borderline
  Compulsive
  Passive-aggressive
	Acting out pattern of behavior
	  Characterized by using socially unacceptable
	  ways of acting out thoughts and feelings

REFERENCES

American Psychiatric Association, 1980. Diagnostic and Statistical Manual of Mental Disorders. 3rd ed. Washington, D.C.

Irving, S., 1983. Basic Psychiatric Nursing. 3rd ed. Philadelphia, W.B. Saunders Co.

Koontz, E., 1982. Schizophrenia: Current diagnostic concepts and implications for nursing care. J Psychosoc Nurs Ment Health Serv, Vol. 20, No. 9, pp. 44–48.

Lipowski, Z.T., 1980. A new look at organic brain syndromes. Am J Psychiatry, Vol. 137, No. 6, June, pp. 674–678.

Mackey, A., 1983. OBS and nursing care. J Gerontol Nurs, Vol. 9, No. 2, February, pp. 74–79, 83–85.

Pavkov, J.R., 1983. Clinical Assessment and Management of the Psychogeriatric Patient. Springhouse, PA, McNeil Pharmaceuticals.

Payne, D., and Clunn, P., 1977. Psychiatric Mental Health Nursing. Garden City, NY, Medical Examination Publishing Company, Inc.

U.S. Department of Health and Human Services, 1981. You Are Not Alone. Rockville, MD, Public Health Service–Alcohol, Drug Abuse, and Mental Health Administration.

4

SPECIFIC PROCESS OF PLANNING CARE

LEARNING OBJECTIVES—Upon completing this chapter, the reader will be able to:

1. Assess a specific individual's strengths, needs, and problems.

2. Develop specific goals that are realistic, measurable, and time-limited and that relate to the individual's needs/problems.

3. List specific approaches and the rationale or reason for using them to achieve the desired goals.

4. Chart the goals that have been set for the individual, using the suggested approaches and showing movement toward the desired goal.

ASSESSMENT OF STRENGTHS, NEEDS, PROBLEMS

The health provider begins planning the client's care by doing an adequate assessment. An assessment is a gathering of comprehensive information about an individual, including what he has going for him (his strengths, needs, or requirements for a reasonable feeling of well-being) and his problems. Such information can be obtained from a variety of sources, including observation, record review, and interview/assessment.

Observations are what you see, hear, and observe about an individual stated as objectively as possible. All subjective (or personal opinions) must be identified as such. Previous records or those that accompany an individual may help in identifying strengths, needs, and problems. The records may also indicate where additional information may be needed. The interview/assessment is a positive and useful tool in gathering needed information from the individual and his support system. A sample Initial Assessment Guide appears at the end of the chapter. The Guide can be adapted or modified according to the health provider's needs.

Finally, all of the information is considered together in identifying the individual's strengths, needs, and problems. This provides the basis for developing specific approaches and realistic and measurable goals.

Strengths are the plusses in an individual's life—what he can do for himself.

Needs, as previously defined, are holes in an individual's life, which, when filled, lead to a reasonable feeling of well-being.

Problems occur when an individual's needs or holes are not adequately filled. The individual experiences or demonstrates difficulty in maintaining stability, which may adversely affect his health, including physical as well as emotional consequences. Problems are listed in the plan of care in the order of their importance. If a problem is considered temporary (i.e., fever, inadequate food and fluid intake, disorientation due to change of environment, abrasions, infections), it should be listed as a *temporary problem* in the plan of care so that it is not overlooked. Temporary problems are short-term problems that resolve within one to six weeks. As temporary problems are resolved, a neat line may be drawn through them so that a permanent record of the individual's problems is maintained. A highlighter pen can sometimes be used so that the resolved problem can be seen more clearly.

SPECIFIC GOALS

Specific goals provide direction for the health provider in caring and planning for the client. They are measurable, attainable, and time-limited achievements or outcomes for the individual. The *focus of goals is on the individual,* not the provider. To get the desired results, a goal must be set for each identified need/problem. Whenever possible, the individual, family, or significant others must participate in the planning of care, including the goal-setting process. The individual's signature, or his guardian's, should appear at the bottom of his care plan to indicate his awareness of what is being done for him.

Goals can be *active goals* or *maintenance goals.* Active goals achieve change/improvement. They can include both long-term and short-term goals.

A *long-term goal* is a general, realistic statement of *hope* for the client. It must be written in terms of what result or outcome will indicate that the need/problem has been resolved. In order to know if there is resolution of the need/problem, the outcome must be observable, measurable, and time-limited. The time element is determined by the policy of the facility. Long-term goals can serve as tools in discharge planning. In deciding on long-term goal issues, keep in mind the growth potential and wishes of the client. Sometimes a long-term goal is referred to simply as the *goal.* Each long term goal should be accompanied by one or more short term goals.

A *short-term goal* is a smaller, more reasonable, and manageable unit of a long-term goal with the same criteria—that is, it specifies the results that are observable, measurable, and time-limited; a time is noted for review and revision. A short-term goal is different from a long-term goal because it is stated in a smaller, manageable unit that is geared to meeting the long-range goal. It is a "bite" of a long-term goal. It defines what can be accomplished in a few days, a week, or a month. A short-term goal is often referred to as the *objective.*

EXAMPLE

Long-term Goal (LTG): Joe Klug will make a decision about where he is going to live within one month (insert date).

Short-term Goal (STG): Mr. Klug will request to talk with his health provider about possible living arrangements outside the institution within two weeks (insert date).

Short-term Goal (STG): Mr. Klug will arrange to visit three possible living arrangements in the community within three weeks (insert date).

A *maintenance goal* is written when improvement is not likely, but where decline is preventable to a large degree. A maintenance goal is self-measuring.

EXAMPLE

Mary Smith's skin over the coccyx area will remain intact. Will be reviewed again on _____
             Month   Year

All goals should be stated *positively* rather than negatively. They should reveal what an individual will be doing rather than what the individual will not do.

EXAMPLE

Positively (right way): Ms. Block will continue taking her daily medication after discharge. To be reviewed _____
(exact date)

Negatively (wrong way): Ms. Block will not stop taking her medication daily after discharge. To be reviewed in one month (exact date).

SPECIFIC APPROACHES

Specific approaches indicate a plan of action that relates directly to the need/problem and offers a possible solution. The possible solution offered should indicate movement toward the desired outcome or goal. Every plan of action should be accompanied by a rationale or reason for using that particular approach. The approaches need to be assigned to the various disciplines that will be implementing them.

The client's identified needs/problems and realistic, measurable, and time-limited goals and approaches make up his *total plan of care*. Other additions to the total plan of care include space for identifying who is responsible for carrying out and reporting progress toward goals and the date of resolution or completion of goals.

A total plan of care means that information from all services providing care to the client is included, such as nursing, dietary, restorative, activity, and social services. Persons representing these services are involved in the planning process, are responsible for implementing the care, and must sign their name on the total plan of care. Most important is that the client be involved in his plan of care at the level at which he can participate and that he sign his care plan if he can understand it and is willing to do so. If the client is unable to sign his plan of care, his personal representative or guardian should review and sign it prior to its implementation.

Each service abstracts from the total plan of care that part of the goal that relates to its specialty. Each service then develops a more detailed plan of care for its staff to use with a particular client. For example, the nursing care plan is a more detailed approach to what nursing staff can do to assist the client in achieving the identified goals in the total plan of care. Since the total plan of care may be part of the permanent record, it should be typed or written in ink.

CHARTING TO THE CARE PLAN

All providers must use the total plan of care as their guide for working with the individual client; therefore, the charting of observations and actions with the client should relate to the client's identified needs/problems, goals, and suggested approaches. It is crucial that the recording show the movement that the client is making toward the stated goals. Data that are new or unrelated to the stated goals, such as vital signs and medications, can be recorded either on flow sheets or in the progress notes according to the facility's protocol.

EXAMPLE OF A TOTAL PLAN OF CARE

Mary Welton is a 70-year-old woman who unpredictably tears anything that she can get hold of—clothing, papers, bedding, etc. She stuffs the things that she tears into her pants. Mary spends her time in the dayroom when she is not tearing. She enjoys catching ball, going outside, playing cards, and sewing.

Strengths: Enjoys playing ball, going outside, playing cards, and sewing.

Revision Date: (Insert exact date—1 month from time written)

DATE	NEED/PROBLEM	ACTIVE GOAL	APPROACH (RATIONALE)
Insert exact date	Rips and tears own and peers' clothing, paper, and magazines about 10 times a day.	Tearing clothing and papers will decrease to 1 time per day in one month. (Insert date)	Unit staff each shift seek out Mary for touch, conversation, and praise when not tearing. (Positive reinforcement) Structure time by increasing number of on and off unit activities, such as playing ball, sewing, walks. (Channeling energy positively) Explain to Mary that her name will be called (i.e., "Mary, no."), everytime she begins to tear. (Limit setting) When Mary responds to cue, "Mary, no," praise her immediately. (Positive reinforcement) Record on flow sheet each time Mary is cued. (Documentation)

DATE	PROGRESS NOTES
Exact Date	*1400—Prob: Tearing clothing; Goal: Decrease tearing*
	Walking about dayroom picking up small pieces of paper from floor. When no one was watching, left the dayroom. Found in another client's room tearing clothes. Stated, "Mary, no." Continued to tear. Took back to dayroom. Involved in game of catch. Tearing decreases if occupied with specific tasks. Tore pieces of clothing six times today. Natalie Dartell, L.P.N.
Exact Date	*1300—Prob: Tearing clothing; Goal: Decrease tearing*
(one week later)	Sewing squares for a quilt today. Praised her for her work. Smiled when she was complimented. Got up to leave the dayroom; staff person said, "Mary, no." Stopped; praised by staff. Indicated had to go to bathroom. Staff went with her. Did tear clothing three times today when no one saw her leave the dayroom. Natalie Dartell, L.P.N.
Exact Date	*2000—Prob: Tearing clothing; Goal: Decrease tearing*
(one week later)	Busy all evening playing cards and sewing. After supper, took a walk with staff. Praised her for participation in card game and help with sewing. Began to enter another client's room. Came back when cue, "Mary, no" was used. Praised by staff. No evidence of tearing this evening. Dawn Powers, L.P.N.

The initial assessment is presented as a method of rapidly assessing the client's immediate physical and mental state at the time of admission. The physical assessment is based on those areas discussed in the section on physical care in Chapter 10. The mental assessment zeroes in on specific presenting problems, many of which are addressed in Chapters 6 and 7. The initial assessment lends itself to the development of a problem list and initial care plan. In this way, the health providers will almost immediately have guidelines for supporting the client in a united manner. Problems to be addressed immediately will be based on the health provider's professional judgment.

INITIAL ASSESSMENT GUIDE

I. PERSONAL DATA

    A. Name _____   Admission Date _____

          Address _____   Phone _____

          _____   Social Security # _____

          Birthdate _____   Age _____ Sex _____

          Religion _____   Race/Culture _____

          Education _____   Occupation _____

          Next of Kin _____   Phone _____

          Address _____   _____

    B. Type of Admission (Voluntary/Involuntary) _____

          Reason for admission (in quotes) _____

          _____

          Presenting Problem _____

          Diagnosis _____

    C. Allergies _____

II. PHYSICAL ASSESSMENT

    A.

	Good	Fair	Poor	Comments
Nutrition				
Elimination				
Sleep and Rest				
Grooming				
Special Problems				

    B. B/P _____ T _____ P _____ R _____ Height _____ Weight _____

    C. Coping Habits: Smoking _____ amt. _____ Alcohol _____ amt. _____

          Prescribed drugs and dosage _____

          Nonprescribed drugs and dosage _____

          Other _____

Interviewer _____

Date of Interview _____

III. MENTAL ASSESSMENT (Check those that apply.)

    A. Perceptions:

          _____ Hallucinations

          _____ Illusions

    B. Thoughts:

          _____ Bizarre thinking or speech   _____ Irrelevancy

          _____ Confusion   _____ Lack of insight

          _____ Defective judgment   _____ Poor concentration

          _____ Delirium   _____ Pressure of speech

          _____ Delusions   _____ Slowed speech

          _____ Disorientation   _____ Somatic concern

          _____ Flight of ideas   _____ Suicidal thoughts

          _____ Grandiosity   _____ Suspiciousness

          _____ Homicidal ideas   _____ Thought disorganization

          _____ Ideas of persecution   _____ Unusual thoughts

          _____ Incoherence

    C. Feelings:

          _____ Anxiety   _____ Guilt feelings

          _____ Apathy (or emotional flatness)   _____ Irritability

          _____ Depressed mood   _____ Feelings of unreality

          _____ Elation

    D. Behavior:

          _____ Aggressiveness   _____ Motor retardation

          _____ Agitation   _____ Negativism

          _____ Assaultiveness   _____ Resistiveness

          _____ Catatonic motor behavior   _____ Social withdrawal

          _____ Deterioration in social habits   _____ Tension

          _____ Facial grimacing   _____ Uncommunicativeness

          _____ Hostility   _____ Uncooperativeness

          _____ Hyperactivity   _____ Withdrawal from reality

          _____ Inappropriateness

INITIAL ASSESSMENT GUIDE— *Continued*

IV. FUNCTIONING AGE _____
V. STRENGTHS _____

VI. SUMMARY _____
_____
_____
_____
_____
_____
_____

Interviewer _____
Date of Interview _____

The initial assessment guide is divided into sections so that it can be completed by two interviewers with different levels of expertise, if desired. Sections I and II include basic personal information and observations regarding the client's immediate physical condition. Sections III, IV, V, and VI call for judgment based on evaluation of what the health provider sees and hears during the interview. Specific observations leading to the conclusions on the initial assessment form are recorded in the client's admission note.

The health provider is encouraged to review the section on communication skills in Chapter 8 as a prelude to the interview and to develop a personal interview technique. Some information will be available from other forms and the client's family. Meanwhile, the following suggestions are offered to the provider:

Rule #1
Simplicity of language is essential!

Rule #2
Read the assessment form prior to going into the interview.

Rule #3
Bring along a blank sheet of paper for notes.

Approach the client in a friendly way. Introduce yourself by name and title. Extend your hand for a handshake. Should the client refuse your hand, simply withdraw your hand without comment—you have already learned something about the client's social interaction with others. Make a statement such as, "I am going to ask you some questions in order to better understand how we can help you during your stay at the center. Please answer to the best of your ability. However, if any of the questions make you feel uncomfortable or you do not wish to answer, please feel free to say so." A good interview is a combination of observation, communication, and knowing when to be silent! Look for nonverbal clues that may contradict the verbal data. Such nonverbal clues often tell you more about the client's thoughts and feelings than his words do.

I. A. Personal data. Although, you may already have this information on another form, asking the questions again is a way to test memory and orientation. Use a lead statement such as, "I know that you have been asked these questions before, but I want to make sure I have the correct information." Have him spell his name. This shows your interest in him and also tests his memory, as do questions about social security number, address, town, and phone number. Playing dumb is an easy way to deal with the date: "Let's see, today's date is

_____." Information about religion indicates whether this is a source of strength for him or the client is involved in a delusional system. Occupation and education also offer information about potential strengths and the level of instruction that will be needed to present new information to the client. "Is there a family member you turn to when you need help? Do we have your permission to contact him during your stay here at the center?" These questions deal with legal issues of client rights and may indicate another strength in the client's life.

B. The client's understanding of his reason for admission is often best obtained by offering an open-ended statement such as, "Obviously, something was not going right for you at home or at work. Tell me about that."

C. Be especially attentive to allergies. Add a word of explanation if needed.

II. A. Physical assessment. At this point, basic, overall information, rather than systems information, is needed. Is the client in immediate physical distress? Look carefully at all the areas that show—hair, skin, eyes, lips, nails, personal hygiene. Ask simple, to-the-point questions about change—what the change is, when it began, and what the client thinks is the reason for the change. Remember to ask if he is on any special diet, either prescribed by the doctor or of his own choice.

B. Coping habits. Find out how much and how often. For example, ask about the client's use of drugs, including prescription, over-the-counter, and street drugs. List each drug's name and the amount the patient takes.

III. A. Mental assessment. Perception comes from the Latin word "perceptio—a gathering together" (Dorland's, 1981:986). The provider must find out how the client is gathering and interpreting sensory data. A question such as "Do you ever see or hear things that other people can not see or hear?" may or may not be answered. Again, observation will offer the provider additional information.

B. Thoughts. Some of this information is obtained while eliciting personal data from the client. For example, by now, the provider should have noted bizarre thoughts or speech, confusion, defective judgment, disorientation, flight of ideas, grandiosity, incoherence, lack of insight, poor concentration, pressure of speech, slowed speech, somatic (bodily) concerns, and thought disorganization. Pointed, simple questions help the provider obtain the rest of the data. For example, "Have you ever had thoughts of hurting yourself? Tell me about it. When was this? Tell me about your plan. What stopped you? Do you still have these feelings?" A similar set of questions is needed in regard to hurting others. "Do you have any enemies who are trying to hurt you? Tell me about it." The client's responses will provide information about suspiciousness and ideas of persecution. "Do you have thoughts that others do not understand? Tell me about them." Throughout the interview, listen intently, and ask additional questions for clarification as needed.

C. Feelings are often easier to evaluate because of the accompanying nonverbal information. "Has anything unpleasant happened to you lately that has changed the way you feel? Tell me about it. Do you sometimes feel sad? Is this more than usual? When did this begin? Do you sometimes feel that you are not really here? Tell me about it. Do you blame yourself for bad things that happen to you or others? Tell me about it." Questions are based on need for more information and clarification.

D. Behavior. Look at the client's nonverbal behavior—his mannerisms, how he sits, stands, walks, gestures, and his accompanying expressions—for clues that will support your observations. Suggested questions include, "Tell me about things that make you angry. What do you do? Does it help?"

IV. Functioning age is based on an assessment of the overall level of functioning. A review of the growth and development chart in Chapter 2 will be helpful. This is valuable information when doing the care plan. Initially, it is impossible for the client to comply past his actual functioning age. The provider and the client will feel less frustrated if this is considered in the plan.

V. Strengths have already been identified, but additional questions may give clues to strengths. For example, "What helps you feel better when you get upset? What activities help you relax? Who helps you most when you get upset?" Remember that ability to care for oneself physically is a strength.

Thank the client for his cooperation. Offer your hand again as you conclude the interview. The notes you have made during the interview will provide the basis for an excellent admission note on the client.

VI. Summaries are usually written according to the protocol of the discipline or institution. The provider is identifying what is going on now for the client and the specific characteristics of this behavior for this client. Take a look at Chapter 5 again.

REFERENCES

Dorland's Illustrated Medical Dictionary, 26th ed. 1981. Philadelphia, W.B. Saunders Co.

The Individualized Planning Training Program. 1980. Richmond, VA. Training and Management Services, Inc.

Joel, L., and Davis, S., 1973. A proposal for baseline data collection for psychiatric care. Perspect Psychiatr Care, Vol. XI, No. 2, pp. 48–58.

Kramer, M., 1972. Nursing care plans—Power to the patient. J Nurs Adm, Vol. II, No. 5, September-October, pp. 29–34.

Mason, A., and Granacher, R., 1980. Clinical Handbook of Anti-Psychotic Drug Therapy. New York, Brunner/Mazel Publishers.

Pfeiffer, E., and Cohen, E., 1983. Assessment: The long term care issues of the '80s. Coordinator, July, pp. 16–17.

Reynolds, J., and Logsdon, J., 1979. Assessing your patient's mental status. Nursing 79, August, pp. 26–33.

Robinson, L., 1983. Psychiatric Nursing As A Human Experience. Philadelphia, W.B. Saunders Co.

Snyder, J., and Wilson, M., 1977. Elements of a Psychological Assessment. Am J Nurs, February, pp. 235–239.

Tyzenhouse, P., 1972. Care Plans for Nursing Home Patients. Nurs Outlook, Vol. 20, No. 3, March, pp. 169–172.

Wagner, B.M., 1969. Care plans—right, reasonable and reachable. Am J Nurs, Vol. 69, No. 5, May, pp. 986–990.

INDEX OF SPECIFIC BEHAVIORS, GOALS, AND APPROACHES

LEARNING OBJECTIVES—Upon completing this chapter, the reader will be able to identify:

1. A long-term goal.

2. A short-term goal.

3. Two approaches for each of the specific problem behaviors presented.

This Chapter is to be used as an **index** for locating behaviors that can present problems. The reason for presenting the behaviors in the chosen format—Need/Problem, Goals, and Approaches—is to give the health provider some direction for working with the specific behavior. **Each behavior must be individualized by listing the specific characteristics that define the behavior for the client.** For ease in locating specific behaviors, the type of behavior will be in bold type in alphabetical order at the left side of the page.

Three core approaches underlie all of the suggested approaches in the index. They are:

1. Help the client identify his problem behavior by using statements such as, "By the way you have been pacing, something seems to be bothering you!"

2. Accept the client as a person without sanctioning his behavior. For example, "You have some good ideas, but I don't approve of your shouting them at me."

3. Explore alternatives and possible consequences for dealing with problem behaviors. For example, "From my observations, the way that you are displaying your anger is getting you into difficulty. Let's talk about other, more acceptable ways that you can deal with your angry feelings."

SPECIFIC BEHAVIORS THAT CAN PRESENT PROBLEMS

GOALS		APPROACH
LONG-TERM GOALS (LTG)	**SHORT-TERM GOALS (STG)**	

AGGRESSIVENESS, PHYSICAL

1. Client will verbalize his problem/needs rather than strike out or fight, within 2 weeks (Insert date)	**a.** Will verbalize signs that indicate he is losing control, within 5 days (Insert date)	The key is *prevention*. Look for signs of mounting tension and intercept by acknowledging the situation (e.g., "I can tell you're irritated.")

GOALS		APPROACH
LONG-TERM GOALS (LTG)	**SHORT-TERM GOALS (STG)**	**APPROACH**

AGGRESSIVENESS, PHYSICAL—*Continued*

		Show genuine concern. Listen and encourage client to speak (e.g., "Go on.") Do not impose your viewpoint. Give client a role in solving the problem. "What would you like us to do?" Set limits on angry behavior. "I'd like you to calm down so I don't have to call for help" (Richardson, Berline-Nauman, 1984:68), or "You do not want to hurt me."

	b. Will inform staff that he is losing control, within 7 days (Insert date)	Basic rules of thumb include:
		  Attitude—calm, friendly, sincere
		  A good-natured sense of humor may get client over a rough spot.
		Don't irritate him. Postpone treatment or routine until he's in a better mood. If an emergency, give client brief explanation, perform treatment quickly with sufficient help, and back off.
		Avoid becoming defensive or angry yourself, since this will only excite client more.
		Avoid arguments.
		Provide enough space for client; keep him away from other clients or visitors who annoy him.
		Do not stand in a doorway. Client may perceive this as being cornered.
		  Stand off to one side in a relaxed position (feet apart to provide a stable base and arms free). Avoid placing hands on hips or making a fist.
		Place objects between you and client (e.g., bed, chair, table).
		Avoid being cornered yourself. Stand on the exit side of the room.
		If client has a dangerous article or is moving at you, throw something at his face for distraction (e.g., sheet, blanket, pillow, garment).
		Remove yourself from the situation as quickly as possible or call for help.

	c. Will go to his room when he thinks that he may be losing control, within 10 days (Insert date)	When client is calm, teach him that he is to go to his room when he thinks he is losing control. Decide on a cue to assist client in following through, such as, "(Client's name), your room."

AGGRESSIVENESS, VERBAL

1. Client will discontinue his verbal aggressiveness and deal with his feelings in a responsible way, such as: —Sublimating through physical activity or hobby.	**a.** Will identify that he has a choice in how he deals with situations and people that provoke verbally aggressive behavior, within 1 week (Insert date)	Collect data base on verbal aggressiveness. Look for signs of mounting tension in the client. Intervene and remind client that he has a choice in how he behaves.

Table continues on following page.

GOALS		APPROACH
LONG-TERM GOALS (LTG)	**SHORT-TERM GOALS (STG)**	

AGGRESSIVENESS, VERBAL—*Continued*

—Removing himself from situations that provoke verbal aggressiveness. —Talking about feelings and emotional reactions without attacking verbally. —Rethinking the situation and changing the way he looks at it, within 6 weeks (Insert date)	**b.** Will identify 4 positive, alternative ways to deal with situations that provoke verbal aggressiveness, within 2 weeks (Insert date)	When client is calm, teach him the problem-solving approach and assist him in looking at new alternative behaviors and their consequences. Remind client that the alternatives he chooses must fit into his life style after discharge. Decide on a cue to assist client in practicing the new alternatives. For example, "(Client's name), stop!"
	c. Will have less than 1 verbal outburst a day, within 3 weeks (Insert date)	Identify specific reinforcers that are dependent upon the number of outbursts and the time involved. When the client has an outburst, ask: —"What did you do?" —"Did it help you or someone else?" —"What are you going to do about it?"

ANGRY FEELINGS, INAPPROPRIATE EXPRESSION OF

1. Client will deal with his angry feelings constructively, through verbalizations and/or physical activity, within 1 month (Insert date)	**a.** Will be able to identify his anger, such as, "I'm angry because my visitors didn't come today," within 1 week (Insert date)	Provide observations on nonverbal behavior to help client identify his anger. Assist client in identifying the source of his anger.
	b. Will automatically go out running when he is angry, within 2 weeks (Insert date)	Provide physical outlets for client's angry feelings.
	c. Will show control over angry feelings by eliminating his destructive behavior, within 3 weeks (Insert date)	Set limits and give positive reinforcement for appropriate behavior.

BLAMING

1. Client will stop blaming others for problems in his life by accepting responsibility for his own behavior, within 6 weeks (Insert date)	**a.** Will identify that he is blaming others for his problems, within 2 weeks (Insert date)	Develop a sincere, nonpunitive relationship with client. Encourage client to ventilate how he feels about certain things. Involve client in assertiveness training.
	b. Will compile a list of his strengths, within 2½ weeks (Insert date)	Assist client in assessing strengths. Encourage client to refer to and add to the list daily. Contact Vocational Services for an in-house job placement.
	c. Will use the problem-solving process as a way of taking responsibility for his behavior, within 5 weeks (Insert date)	Teach client the problem-solving process. (Refer to Chapter 2.) Reinforce new behaviors verbally and through special privileges that are important to the client.

DELUSIONS THAT INTERFERE WITH FUNCTIONING

1. Client will control his delusional behavior so that	**a.** Will stop talking about his delusions, within 2 weeks	Do not agree or disagree with client's delusions. Calmly and quietly communicate that you do

GOALS		APPROACH
LONG-TERM GOALS (LTG)	**SHORT-TERM GOALS (STG)**	

DELUSIONS THAT INTERFERE WITH FUNCTIONING—*Continued*

his delusions will not interfere with his role performance, such as carrying out his activities of daily living, within 4 weeks (Insert date)	(Insert date)	understand what he might be experiencing at the time but it is not real. Divert his attention by involving him in simple activity. Set limits, if necessary, on discussion of delusions. For example, "You do not benefit from this topic of discussion" (Payne, 1977:90), or "If you want to stay out of the hospital, you have to stop talking about these ideas that aren't true."
	b. Will respond to the following statement: "What is it that you wanted and went about getting in a way that others did not approve of that resulted in your hospitalizataion?" within 3 weeks (Insert date)	Help client identify his needs and ways to meet them. Do not permit anyone to make fun of client.

DEMANDING

1. Client will make legitimate requests of staff, as for money to go shopping, rather than unreasonable demands, as for bringing him food from the canteen when he could do it himself, within 6 months (Insert date)	**a.** Demands of staff will decrease, as reflected in the data base, as staff spend more time with client when he is not demanding, within 1 month (Insert date)	Determine what needs client is trying to fulfill through his demands. Spend time with client when he is not demanding.
	b. Will increase the tasks that he can do by and for himself, within 3 months (Insert date)	Help identify one thing client can do by and for himself.

DENIAL

1. Client will accept the reality of his present situation, such as the loss of a loved one, illness, alcoholism, within 6 weeks (Insert date)	**a.** Will actively participate in identifying the problem and exploring alternatives to his situation, within 2 weeks (Insert date)	Establish meaning of situation for client and convey to him that he can move through it.
	b. Will select and implement an alternative to his situation, within 4 weeks (Insert date)	Teach client problem-solving process: —Identify the problem. —Explore several alternatives and possible consequences. —Choose the best alternative. —Evaluate the consequence. —If not successful, repeat process.
	c. Will evaluate the effectiveness of the alternative that he chose and pursue need for further action, within 5 weeks (Insert date)	

DISROBING

1. Client will keep his clothes	**a.** Will keep his clothes on	Collect data base on disrobing—frequency and

Table continues on following page.

GOALS		APPROACH
LONG-TERM GOALS (LTG)	**SHORT-TERM GOALS (STG)**	

DISROBING—*Continued*

on during the waking hours, by the end of 2 months (Insert date)	while he is involved in activities, within 2 weeks (Insert date)	precipitating factors. Dress client in comfortable clothes that fit well and look as nice as possible. Fix client's clothes so that he cannot remove them easily (choose clothes that open at the back). Make a structured plan to keep the client busy with useful or pleasant work and games. Protect the client from being embarrassed, exposed, or ridiculed. Check client frequently and redress as needed, without comment. Attitude is important. Be matter-of-fact. Client must not be punished or shamed.

DISTRESSFUL BEHAVIOR THAT INTERFERES WITH FUNCTIONING

1. Client will use positive ways to relieve distress that he can incorporate into his life style, within 6 weeks (Insert date) (List specific positive ways appropriate for the behavior.)	**a.** Will practice 2 ways that have been helpful in the past to reduce his distress, within 1 week (Insert date) **b.** Will practice 1 additional new way of dealing with distress, within 2 weeks (Insert date)	Encourage client to verbalize his feelings. Explore with client past solutions that have been helpful. Support client in practicing old, successful ways of relieving distress that are healthy and appropriate in the setting. Assess with client his practices regarding: —Nutrition —Work habits —Sources of satisfaction —Relaxation —Exercises —Recreation —Rest —Need for information to deal with special stressors, such as finances, interpersonal relationships, assertiveness Structure client's day to involve him in appropriate information classes, groups, or one-on-one sessions about topics identified in previous step so that he learns new ways of dealing with his particular distress. Praise client for following plan.

EATING, REFUSAL

1. Client will voluntarily eat his meals, within 1 month (Insert date)	**a.** Will eat his meals with assistance, within 5 days (Insert date)	Talk pleasantly and quietly to the client. Don't criticize client's eating habits or make a fuss about the additional attention he needs. Remember not to rush client. Seat client next to a client who eats readily. If this does not work, offer a tray on the unit. Encourage client to eat. Talk about building up physically to get well and go home. Present small portions. Limit choices of food on tray. Help client cut and prepare his food. Assist only as needed, using a spoon. Sometimes

GOALS		APPROACH
LONG-TERM GOALS (LTG)	**SHORT-TERM GOALS (STG)**	

EATING, REFUSAL—*Continued*

		putting food on the spoon will be enough to encourage client to continue eating. You may need to fill the spoon, put it in his hand, and have him continue feeding himself. If necessary, feed him a few spoonfuls and encourage him to continue. Spoon-feed completely only if client is unable to do so with partial assistance.
	b. Will eat 50 per cent of his meal by himself, within 2 weeks (Insert date)	Reinforce desired behavior. Client must not be scolded or punished for not eating. Do not threaten the client to force eating. *Do not* force-feed. Client will not digest the food well and may *aspirate*. Weigh client daily. Keep doctor informed in case additional measures are necessary.

FORGETFULNESS RESULTING FROM ORGANIC BRAIN IMPAIRMENT

1. Client will be receptive to methods that will help him remember, within 2 months (Insert date)	**a.** Will add information about his past to conversation initiated by staff, within 2 weeks (Insert date)	Refrain from asking questions client cannot answer. Discuss events from the past that client can share. Use the client's experiences in the past to orient him to the present. (Refer to Chapter 9.) If client has forgotten recent events that you know about, help him answer questions correctly. Protect client from embarrassment. Do not let other clients tease him.
	b. Will recognize his name in large print on his room, by the end of 1 month (Insert date)	Begin compiling a list of recent events that client can refer to, to help him remember. Use calendars, clocks, bulletin boards and labels with client's name to reinforce his memory. The client's name in large print will help him find his room. Color-coding will help the client identify his belongings.

GUILTY FEELING, INAPPROPRIATE USE OF

1. Client will identify the constructive alternative that relieves the feeling of guilt, within 6 months (Insert date)	**a.** Will be able to verbalize when his feeling of guilt started, within 2 weeks (Insert date)	Determine the appropriateness of need to feel guilty by exploring source. Avoid reinforcing, verbally and/or nonverbally, the client's belief that he is guilty.
	b. Will be able to identify that he is angry when he says, "I'm guilty," within 3 months (Insert date)	When client says, "I'm guilty," ask him to substitute the words, "I'm angry" or "I resent it," or ask client how long he needs to punish himself. Then, set a time limit for client to indulge in his guilty feelings. Fade out the guilty behavior by gradually decreasing the allotted time for the behavior and increasing the client's involvement outside self, such as assisting with simple chores in the unit.

Table continues on following page.

GOALS		
LONG-TERM GOALS (LTG)	**SHORT-TERM GOALS (STG)**	**APPROACH**

HALLUCINATIONS THAT INTERFERE WITH FUNCTIONING

1. The client will be able to control his hallucinations and respond to the real environment, within 4 weeks (Insert date)	**a.** Will admit to the presence of hallucinations, within 1 week (Insert date)	Have client name the fact that he is anxious or lonely, and connect the hallucinating behavior to it. This will help provide control over hallucinatory process. Develop a one-to-one relationship with client. Discuss real events with client; focus on reality. Refer to voices as "so-called voices." Do not act attentive to discussion regarding hallucinations. This will decrease importance of hallucinations.
	b. Will follow direction for temporary relief of hallucinations, within 2 weeks (Insert date)	Suggest an activity, such as singing, when client hears voices, to provide temporary relief of the hallucinations.
	c. Will dismiss voices, within 3 weeks (Insert date)	Teach client to dismiss the hallucinations. For example, instruct client to tell voices to "Go away" or "Leave me alone." Reassure client and provide additional attention from staff during this time.

HELPLESSNESS

1. Client will deal with feelings of helplessness constructively by doing things that he had depended on others to do, within 6 weeks (Insert date) (List specific areas in which client will become independent.)	**a.** Will be able to identify use of helplessness and verbalize the reason, such as "I can't be like you, but I can force you to take care of me," or "If I can't do it my way, I won't do anything," within 3 weeks (Insert date)	Provide feedback on client's behavior, both verbal and nonverbal, to help client identify use of helplessness. Initiate discussion of the underlying feeling experienced prior to use of helplessness (e.g., anger, jealousy, fear). Teach client basics of assertiveness through assertiveness group twice a week.
	b. Will show control over helplessness by doing the activity that he previously would have avoided, within 4 weeks (Insert date)	Help identify 1 thing daily that client can do by and for himself. (Review in 2 weeks.) Reinforce independent behavior verbally. Initiate discussion about how client feels when he follows through with activity.

HOARDING

1. The client will stop hoarding (specific items), within 3 months (Insert date)	**a.** Will stop acquiring the hoarded item himself, within 1 month (Insert date)	Collect data base on frequency and amount of hoarding. Move all previously hidden items into client's room. Inform client that he will receive a specific number of items daily. State exact number. Direct client to keep all items in his room and not throw or give any away. Count items daily to be sure they are not being discarded.
	b. Will request that the items be removed from his room, within 2½ months (Insert date)	Continue to increase the supply in the predetermined manner until the client requests that all items be removed from his room. However, if the hoarded items include food or potentially harmful items such as metal or glass, implement other measures. For example, explain to client that hoarding

GOALS		APPROACH
LONG-TERM GOALS (LTG)	**SHORT-TERM GOALS (STG)**	

HOARDING—*Continued*

		food is unsanitary, since it attracts bugs. Reassure client that he will receive plenty of food. Allow him to keep enough for an evening snack.
		Regular cleaning with client is necessary. Be honest with the client when you take the extra food away. He has the right to know where his possessions are, and even though he doesn't like what you're doing, he will trust you more.

IDEAS OF REFERENCE THAT INTERFERE WITH FUNCTIONING

1. Client will dismiss casual remarks or behaviors as not applying to him, within 6 weeks (Insert date)	**a.** Will ask for confirmation of what he is hearing, within 3 weeks (Insert date)	Reassure client that verbalization or behavior does not apply to him. For example, "No, the police officer is not here to get you. He brought a new client to the unit."
	b. Will identify that he used to believe that remarks or behaviors applied to him, within 5 weeks (Insert date)	Reassure client that his ideas of reference are part of his illness, and his ability to say that he "used to believe" shows that he is improving.

ILLUSIONS THAT INTERFERE WITH FUNCTIONING

1. Client will be able to correctly identify what he sees and hears, within 10 days (Insert date)	**a.** Will begin to question his illusions, within 5 days (Insert date)	Be honest with client. Describe carefully what he is looking at or listening to, and explain honestly what it really is. Do not let others fool or frighten him. Avoid arguments. Keep client occupied with work or activities. Be calm and reassuring. The client needs to know that this is part of his illness that will subside as he continues to improve.

IMPULSIVENESS

1. Client will talk through his problems rather than act on his feelings, within 6 weeks (Insert date)	**a.** Will verbalize factors that trigger his behavior, within 3 weeks (Insert date)	Collect data on frequency and precipitating factors of impulsive behavior. Point out the consequences of impulsive acts.
	b. Will request assistance in maintaining control, within 4 weeks (Insert date)	Interrupt any impulsive act and explore alternative behaviors. Teach client to identify thoughts and feelings before acting on feelings.

INABILITY TO FOLLOW DIRECTIONS

1. Client will follow directions using written directions as a reminder, within 2 weeks (Insert date)	**a.** Will follow directions when directions are given prior to activity, within 1 week (Insert date)	Address client by name. Be sure you have his attention. Speak quietly in a low, firm voice. Be unhurried and reassuring. Use statements rather than questions, using "I" instead of "you." For example, "I want you to go for a walk with me," instead of "You should go for a walk." Be direct. Use short, simple, to-the-point sentences.

Table continues on following page.

GOALS		APPROACH
LONG-TERM GOALS (LTG)	**SHORT-TERM GOALS (STG)**	

INABILITY TO FOLLOW DIRECTIONS—*Continued*

		Give directions prior to activity.
		Ask the client to restate what you have told him to do.
		Give client written schedule/instructions to support verbal instructions. Observe behavior. If client does not comply, refer him to written schedule and review it with him.
		Prompt client as needed. Make brief, frequent contacts throughout the day. Ask for and answer questions.
		Reinforce client verbally when he follows directions.

INDECISIVENESS

1. Client will make basic decisions, such as what to eat, what to wear, what activities to engage in, by himself, within 1 month (Insert date)	**a.** Will identify each decision-making step he gets stuck on, within 2 weeks (Insert date)	Instruct client regarding what to do as a way of teaching new responses. Using the problem-solving process, explore with client the level at which he has difficulty making a decision. (Refer to Chapter 2.)
	b. Will make a decision when offered two choices, within 3 weeks (Insert date)	Reassure the client that it is O.K. to make a decision and to be wrong. Offer the client two choices. (Be careful not to choose for him.) Praise him for making a choice. Insist that the client follow through on the choice he has made. Reinforce positively client's success in decision making and follow through. Reinforcers must be predetermined and of significance to client.

INSTITUTIONALIZED BEHAVIOR

1. Client will live in a less restrictive setting, such as a halfway house, within 1 year (Insert date)	**a.** Will perform his personal care skills with supervision, within 3 months (Insert date). (This goal would be revised until client performs these tasks without supervision.)	Help identify areas client can control, using a behavior modification approach with positive reinforcement. Teach client basic skills, such as bathing, care of clothing, table manners.
	b. Will approach another client and initiate an activity, within 4 months (Insert date). (This goal would be revised to move from a one-on-one relationship into a group situation.)	Through social skills training, teach client to actively participate in his care.

LONELINESS, FEELINGS OF, THAT INTERFERE WITH FUNCTIONING

1. Client will deal with feelings of loneliness by continuing group activities and developing a relationship with one other client,	**a.** Will develop a relationship with one assigned staff member, within 1 week (Insert date)	Develop a relationship with client. Begin with short, frequent visits. Always address client respectfully, by name. Use touch—shoulders, hand, wrist, or arm—to convey empathy.

GOALS		APPROACH
LONG-TERM GOALS (LTG)	**SHORT-TERM GOALS (STG)**	

LONELINESS, FEELINGS OF, THAT INTERFERE WITH FUNCTIONING—*Continued*

within 3 weeks (Insert date)		Be alert to your own feelings of loneliness, and do not confuse them with client's. Discuss with client reason for present loneliness—choice, circumstances, or lack of knowledge on how to make contacts.
	b. Will attend regularly scheduled activities, within 2 weeks (Insert date)	Explore previous successful ways client dealt with loneliness. Plan a regular schedule of activities with client that he will attend, including occupational therapy and social therapeutic group. Initially attend activities with client, and initiate involvement. Request client to assist with useful activities, such as watering flowers, passing trays. Encourage client to seek out one other client whom he likes, and initiate one daily activity with him. Listen to client talk about his feelings. Reinforce desired behavior. Discuss other possible contacts, such as involvement in church, volunteer activities.

MANIPULATION, DESTRUCTIVE

1. Client will eliminate his exploitation of others, such as "playing one staff member against another," within 1 year (Insert date)	**a.** Will demonstrate self-control of his behavior by not having to be reminded of his limits, within 4 months (Insert date)	Discuss with client the cause and effect of his behavior in relation to his environment. Be consistent and firm with limits set on client's behavior and with expectations and consequences communicated to client and staff. Provide verbal and nonverbal reinforcement when client functions within the limits placed on his behavior.
	b. Will realistically plan his activities for the day and adhere to his schedule, within 8 months (Insert date)	Teach client to plan daily activities and to concentrate on following plan.

MASTURBATION IN PUBLIC PLACES

1. Client will discontinue masturbating in public, within 6 months (Insert date)	**a.** Will go to his room to masturbate with cuing such as, "Joe, go to your room," within 3 months (Insert date)	Identify situations in which masturbation occurs. Give feedback to client about the uncomfortableness that his public masturbation creates in others.
	b. Will go to his room without cuing, within 5 months (Insert date)	Discuss and negotiate ways to provide privacy (e.g., in his room with the door closed).

MISIDENTIFICATION THAT INTERFERES WITH FUNCTIONING

1. Client will call people (or objects) by their correct	**a.** Will begin to question his misidentifications (include	Briefly and matter-of-factly tell client correct name of person (or object).

Table continues on following page.

GOALS		APPROACH
LONG-TERM GOALS (LTG)	**SHORT-TERM GOALS (STG)**	

MISIDENTIFICATION THAT INTERFERES WITH FUNCTIONING—*Continued*

name, within 3 weeks (Insert date)	specifics), within 2 weeks (Insert date)	Avoid arguments with client about his misidentification. Avoid answering to an incorrect name. Tell client what your real name is and answer to that name. Be patient and tactful in dealing with client. Prevent other clients from stimulating client's misidentification.

NOCTURNAL WANDERING

1. Client will go back to sleep after awakening at night, within 2 weeks (Insert date)	**a.** Will decrease wandering pattern by half, as identified in the data base, within 10 days (Insert date)	Collect data base on frequency of wandering. Evaluate changes that may indicate a physical problem, such as cold, flu, or organic impairment. Identify whether client has a problem/need, such as: —the need to go to the bathroom —incontinence —cold —hunger —boredom —anxiety —disorientation Deal with the specific problem/need. Use basic nursing techniques to settle patient. For example, —tighten sheets —provide extra blanket —provide small snack or warm milk —give back rub with warmed lotion —sit with client —reassure client —reorient client, as needed —provide night light or additional light, as needed If necessary, —permit wandering within safe area. —involve client in subdued activities. —permit client to rest in an easy chair close to unit station. Continue to use the above mentioned basic nursing techniques nightly, focusing on most successful combination.

NONASSERTIVENESS

1. Client will respond honestly to what he does or does not want to do when requests are made, within 4 weeks (Insert date)	**a.** Will identify the underlying feelings experienced when doing something he does not want to do, within 1 week (Insert date)	Interest client in beginning a "Doormat (Poor Me) Journal," and note incidents that happened throughout the day. Suggest 4 columns, called: —What happened —Outcome (including feelings) —What I really wanted to do —What stopped me Review the journal once daily with staff.

GOALS		APPROACH
LONG-TERM GOALS (LTG)	**SHORT-TERM GOALS (STG)**	**APPROACH**

NONASSERTIVENESS—*Continued*

		Direct client to attend weekly assertiveness group sessions.
	b. Will succeed in saying "No" to requests that he does not want to do and "Yes" to requests he wants to do 50% of time, within 2 weeks (Insert date). (This goal would be revised until client is able to say "No" without feeling guilty.)	Direct client to practice desired responses by writing them down. Direct client to monitor his responses throughout the day on the form provided. Identify specific reinforcers for 50% success; continue on up to 100% success.

NONCOMPLIANCE

1. Client will follow through with his structured plan of care (include areas of compliance needed), within 4 weeks (Insert date)	**a.** Will contribute to a care plan that includes some of his choices, within 1 week (Insert date)	Attitude is important. Project that you believe client wants to comply. Explain in detail the importance of complying with his treatment plan, the consequences involved, and the options available. Assess client's needs for his age, growth, and development level. (Refer to section on the Young, Chronically Ill Client.) Assign staff consistently to work with client and develop a relationship.
	b. Will follow a structured, daily plan and receive reinforcers for compliance as specified in the plan, within 2 weeks (Insert date)	Encourage client to talk about his personal plan. Provide feedback on what is realistic at this time. Develop a structured, daily plan and incorporate client's choices as much as possible. Review plan with client. Give him a copy. Have client attend classes on special needs, such as money management, medication, cooking. List specific positive reinforcers for compliance. Contact the follow-up worker for continued support and assistance to client after discharge.

PHYSICAL SYMPTOMS, INAPPROPRIATE USE OF

1. Client will deal with his emotional needs constructively, such as getting involved in volunteer work, within 6 weeks (Insert date)	**a.** Will express how he feels rather than focus on his physical symptoms, within 3 weeks (Insert date)	Collect data on the character, duration, and frequency of symptoms.
	b. Will use relaxation techniques as a way of handling his anxiety, within 4 weeks (Insert date)	Teach client about people's basic emotional needs and ways they are met.
	c. Will assist staff with small tasks, such as folding laundry, within 5 weeks (Insert date)	Focus on client when he is symptom-free, and redirect his attention outside self.

Table continues on following page.

GOALS		
LONG-TERM GOALS (LTG)	SHORT-TERM GOALS (STG)	APPROACH

SECLUSIVENESS THAT INTERFERES WITH FUNCTIONING

1. Client will join group activities on his own, within 3 weeks (Insert date)	**a.** Will accept one-to-one contact with assigned staff, within 10 days (Insert date)	Approach client on one-to-one basis for short periods of time. Talk about neutral topics and any topics in which he shows interest. Lengthen contacts as tolerated by client. Invite client to play a game or participate in an activity with you. Initiate conversation about whom he has noticed on the unit and in whom he has some interest.
	b. Will join group activities when invited by peers or staff, within 2 weeks (Insert date)	Invite client to watch a group activity. Casually invite him to join. Reassure him if he seems tense, and encourage him to complete the activity. Praise him for his participation and accomplishment.

SEXUAL ACTING OUT

1. Client will eliminate inappropriate sexual behavior, within 4 weeks (Insert date)	**a.** Will verbalize situations in which his sexual acting out behavior occurs, within 2 weeks (Insert date)	Identify situations in which sexual acting out occurs.
	b. Upon cuing, such as suggesting an activity, client will discontinue inappropriate sexual behavior, within 3 weeks (Insert date)	Openly discuss sexual behavior, and clarify any misconceptions about staff/client relationships. Teach client appropriate ways of dealing with sexual impulses.

SLEEP, UNSATISFIED

1. Client will return to previous satisfying pattern of sleep, within 3 weeks (Insert date)	**a.** Will identify his usual sleep pattern and needs, within 2 days (Insert date)	Monitor and record client's rest and sleep pattern for 2 days. Listen to client discuss his usual sleep pattern and sleep need. Provide feedback to client regarding your observation of his rest and sleep pattern.
	b. Will identify the kinds of situations that promote or prevent sleep for him, within 4 days (Insert date)	Discuss with client his previous pre-bedtime activities. Discuss with client any changes in pre-bedtime pattern and when the changes began.
	c. Will implement methods to induce sleep, within 1 week (Insert date)	Reassure client that it is O.K. not to sleep. Have client refrain from eating shortly before bedtime. Direct client to take a 20-minute bubble bath prior to bedtime. Offer client a backrub after bath. Direct client to follow directions on relaxation tape, being careful to avoid sleeping. Have client continue this ritual nightly, beginning at the same time each evening.

GOALS		APPROACH
LONG-TERM GOALS (LTG)	**SHORT-TERM GOALS (STG)**	

SLEEP, UNSATISFIED—*Continued*

		Instruct client to get up immediately upon awakening from sleep, rather than staying in bed.

TATTLING

1. Client will deal directly with significant individuals, rather than tattling, within 4 weeks (Insert date)	**a.** Will deal directly with individual concerned when accompanied by a staff person, within 2 weeks (Insert date)	Interrupt the behavior. Explain to client what you observed happening. Give client the following information: —"I will not deal with the problem you are having with (specific name). However, I will go with you when you talk to her about this problem. I will be your silent support." —If client is unsure how to handle problem, offer the following: —Talk to (specific name) about the feeling you are experiencing in response to what happened. —Use "I" centered statements. For example, "I was hurt when you said that I am stupid."
	b. Will identify feelings experienced with use of confrontation, within 3 weeks (Insert date)	Encourage ventilation by having client regard the confrontation in terms of: —risk —feelings —value to client and individual involved Praise client for successful follow-through.

TEMPER TANTRUMS

1. Client will replace temper tantrums with a constructive way of expressing self, within 2 months (Insert date)	**a.** Will limit his temper tantrums to half the number per day, identified in the data base, within 1 month (Insert date)	Collect data base on temper tantrums. Review behavioral guidelines and consequences with client, (e.g., a 2 minute time-out, or, if client cannot take time-out, staff will hold him). Give client a copy of guidelines. Make a list of the positive reinforcers client can receive for no time-outs and for certain number of time-outs. Give client a copy.
	b. Will identify reason for tantrums, within 6 weeks (Insert date)	Develop a trusting relationship with client. Ask client to identify reason for behavior.
	c. Will go to his room and play his drums instead of having a tantrum, within 7 weeks (Insert date)	Discuss alternative behaviors with client when he is calm. Cue client if necessary, to go to his room. Say "(Client's name), room."

WORRY, INAPPROPRIATE EXPRESSION OF

1. Client will give up constant worrying about situations he cannot control, within 6 months (Insert date)	**a.** Will determine which worries are past or future and those for which others are responsible, within 2	Listen to client discuss his worries. Have him begin a "worry journal" where he sorts his worries into the following categories: past, future, others' responsibility, and

Table continues on following page.

GOALS		APPROACH
LONG-TERM GOALS (LTG)	**SHORT-TERM GOALS (STG)**	

WORRY, INAPPROPRIATE EXPRESSION OF—*Continued*

	months (Insert date)	legitimately his own. Review the journal daily with client.
	b. Will discuss feelings experienced when attempting not to worry, within 3 months (Insert date)	Listen to client express the feelings he experiences. Reassure him that this is to be expected.
	c. Will sign a limited worry contract, within 4 months (Insert date)	Discuss the contract with the client, as follows: —Determine if the worry belongs to him and if it is in the present. —If the worry does not belong to him, have him record it in his journal and refuse to worry about it. Tell him to use reminders such as, "That worry does not belong to me!" —If the worry is in the present, have client determine how much time he needs for worrying; then tell him to limit himself to this amount of time. —Suggest reminders to control returning worry such as "I've already worried long enough about you!" —Gradually decrease the amount of time client uses for worrying about any issue. —Advise client to postpone realistic worry that belongs in the future with reminders such as, "I'll worry about the results of the tests next Friday when I go to see the doctor again." (If necessary, post such dates on a calendar and insist that the client not worry about them until the actual day.) —Review progress with client weekly. Gradually increase the time between reviews.

REFERENCES

Berkowitz, L., 1971. The case for bottling up rage. Psychol Today, July, pp. 24–31.

Brunner, L.S., 1982. Lippincott's Manual of Nursing. 3rd ed. Philadelphia, Lippincott Publishing Co.

Field, W., and Ruelka, W., 1973. Hallucinations and how to deal with them. Am J Nurs, Vol. 73, No. 4, April, pp. 638–640.

Glasser, W., 1965. Reality Therapy. New York, Harper and Row Publishers, Inc.

Knowles, R., 1982. Managing angry feelings. Am J Nurs, Vol. 82, No. 21, February, p. 299.

Le Shan, E., 1983. Beware the helpless. Woman's Day, April 26, pp. 50–52.

Menninger, C., Edmundson, R., and Johnson, B. Aid for Better Understanding of Mentally Ill.

Payne, D., and Clunn, P., 1977. Psychiatric Mental Health Nursing. 2nd ed. New York, Medical Examination Publishing Company, Inc.

Perko, J., and Kreigh, H., 1983. Psychiatric and Mental Health Nursing: A Commitment to Care and Concern. 2nd ed. Virginia, Reston Publishing Company, Inc.

Powell, J., 1969. Why Am I Afraid to Tell You Who I Am? Niles, IL., Argus Communications.

Richardson, J., and Berline-Nauman, D., 1984. The face of anger. Nursing '84, February, pp. 66–71.

Smith, C., and Murphy, K., 1984. Developing a children's inpatient psychiatric unit. J Psychosocial Nurs, Vol. 22, No. 3, March, pp. 31–36.

Veterans Administration, 1972. Program guide. Washington, DC, April 28.

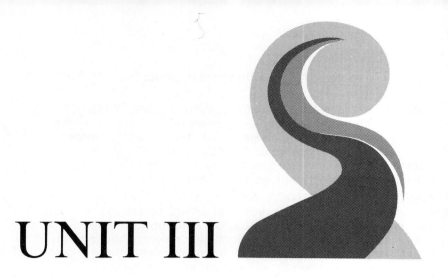

UNIT III

SPECIFIC PATTERNS OF BEHAVIOR WITH SAMPLE PLANS OF CARE

When working with emotionally disturbed clients, distinct patterns of behavior must be identified. For presentation purposes, each pattern will be dealt with individually. However, every client is different, so behavior patterns may overlap, or a client may exhibit more than one behavior pattern at various times during the period in which the health provider is giving care.

With each specific pattern of behavior presented in Chapters 6, 7, 8, and 9, a "Description" of the behavior will be provided, including coping/mental mechanisms used and suggested "Interventions." A sample plan of care for a hypothetical client with the particular behavior follows. These sample plans of care are, of course, only *guidelines*. The plan of care the health provider develops must be tailored to meet each client's specific needs/problems. References that might be helpful in planning care for clients with the specific patterns of behavior discussed can be found at the end of this unit.

The format to be followed in presenting the plans of care will focus on the core of the plan of care: strengths, needs/problems, approach, and realistic, measurable, and time-limited goals.

STRENGTHS: What are the pluses in the client's life? What does he have going for him? What can he do for himself that the health provider can utilize in planning his care?

NEEDS/PROBLEMS: What are the areas in the client's life that are interfering with his ability to care for himself, both physically and mentally? The areas that require attention should be listed in the form of a statement.

REALISTIC, MEASURABLE, AND TIME-LIMITED GOALS: These goals refer to measurable and attainable client achievements. Whenever possible, the client, family, or significant others must participate in the planning of care. These goals must be revised at regularly scheduled intervals, depending on changes in the client's condition. These revision times must be noted on the plan of care.

APPROACH, INTERVENTION, STRATEGY, SOLUTION: These terms indicate a specific plan of action that relates directly to the identified needs/problems and offer a possible solution to the need/problem. With every plan of action, a rationale or reason should be given for using that particular approach. In the plans of care that are presented in this book, the rationale will appear in parentheses.

SPECIFIC PATTERNS OF BEHAVIOR RELATED TO THE MAJOR MENTAL DISORDERS

LEARNING OBJECTIVES—Upon completing this chapter, the reader will be able to:

1. Give two identifying characteristics for the withdrawal pattern of behavior, overly suspicious pattern of behavior, depressive pattern of behavior, overactive (manic) pattern of behavior, suicidal pattern of behavior, and behavior patterns of the young, chronically mentally ill.

2. List two significant interventions for each of the patterns of behavior discussed.

WITHDRAWAL PATTERN OF BEHAVIOR

DESCRIPTION

The withdrawal pattern of behavior is usually seen in those people who are suffering from schizophrenic disorders.

Clients with withdrawal patterns of behavior may have been exposed to a great deal of conflict and turmoil during their early developmental periods. As a result of these early experiences they never fully develop a basic sense of trust. They continue throughout life to search for acceptance and approval. After numerous rejections, they eventually give up, and, utilizing the coping/mental mechanism of *regression,* retreat to a simpler form of existence in a world of their own. In this world, they turn their attention to themselves and relate to their imaginary environment as if it were real.

One of the most pronounced difficulties these persons have is the inability to relate in a meaningful way to other people. To avoid further rejection, they set up barriers that make it difficult for persons to establish contact. For the health provider, these barriers are obstacles to the establishment of a trusting relationship.

Below the surface is a very lonely and frightened person who desperately wants someone to care for him. His loneliness and fear are evident in his distorted thoughts, feelings, and actions. The distortions vary and may include delusions, hallucinations, flat or inappropriate affect, socially unacceptable behavior, and ambivalence. Ambivalence in particular presents many problems because the individual experiences, at the same time, opposing feelings toward the same object, person, or idea, and the opposing feelings interfere with his decision-making.

INTERVENTIONS

When working with persons who have a withdrawal pattern of behavior, remember two important approaches. First, initiate contact on a one-to-one basis. Second, meet the clients at their level of functioning. Be sensitive to the clues clients provide, such as their need for personal space and their inability to engage in meaningful conversation. For example, it may be helpful to say, "If you would rather not talk, I'll just sit here for 10 minutes." A time limit structures the interaction. The client develops trust when he sees you doing what you said you would do.

The health provider must be patient when working with withdrawn clients. A rejection from such a client is often a clue that he has allowed the health provider to enter his world. However, the entrance may have made the client uncomfortable. The health provider should not view this as a permanent rejection by the client. Instead, he should move more slowly. The withdrawn client cannot tolerate criticism or judgment from his caretakers. He needs a supportive health provider who will make no demands. Because he is afraid to trust, developing the relationship will be a slow process.

The Essential Components of a Plan of Care for a Client with a Withdrawal Pattern of Behavior

Miss Shari Hall, age 20, has fine features, fair skin, and long, ash-blond hair. She spends the day sitting on the floor in the corner of the dayroom with her arms clasped about her knees. When she is alone, she will laugh for no apparent reason, turn her head to the side as though listening to someone, and respond with lengthy conversations that seem meaningless but indicate a good vocabulary. Because she is so preoccupied, she neglects her physical care. She can be distracted from her preoccupation if approached in a warm and casual way.

THE ESSENTIAL COMPONENTS OF A PLAN OF CARE FOR A CLIENT WITH A WITHDRAWAL PATTERN OF BEHAVIOR

STRENGTHS: Miss Shari Hall's attractiveness, good vocabulary, and response to being approached				Revision Date: Insert date
DATE	**NEED/PROBLEM**	**GOALS**		**APPROACH**
		LONG-TERM GOALS (LTG)	**SHORT-TERM GOALS (STG)**	
Insert date	1. Loss of contact with reality.	1. Shari Hall will maintain contact with reality daily during her waking hours, within 3 weeks (Insert date)	a. Will allow health provider to sit near her 3 times a day for 5-minute intervals without getting up and leaving, within 4 days (Insert date)	Give medication as ordered. (Decrease symptoms.) Approach Shari for short intervals without expecting her to talk to you. Let her know that it's O.K. to be silent. (Decrease anxiety of your presence.)
			b. Will go for a walk with the health provider 2 times a day, within 10 days (Insert date)	Distract Shari from her preoccupation by approaching her in a warm, friendly way to take a walk. (Environment is one way of focusing on reality.)
			c. Will participate in a game of Scrabble with the health provider, within 2 weeks (Insert date)	Suggest playing a game of Scrabble with Shari on a one-on-one basis. (Opportunity to use her strength of a good vocabulary in a realistic way.)
			d. Will participate in a game of Scrabble with the health provider and another	Temporary rejections of the health provider are not to be taken personally. They are the client's way of testing

THE ESSENTIAL COMPONENTS OF A PLAN OF CARE FOR A CLIENT WITH A WITHDRAWAL PATTERN OF BEHAVIOR—*Continued*

STRENGTHS: Miss Shari Hall's attractiveness, good vocabulary, and response to being approached

Revision Date: Insert date

DATE	NEED/PROBLEM	GOALS		APPROACH
		LONG-TERM GOALS (LTG)	**SHORT-TERM GOALS (STG)**	
			client, within 2½ weeks (Insert date)	you to see if you can be trusted.
			e. Will initiate activities with health provider and other clients, within 3 weeks (Insert date)	Encourage Shari to choose a client to join your game of Scrabble. Assign Shari the task of initiating an activity.
Insert date	**2.** Neglects physical care, including eating, bathing, hair care, oral hygiene.	**2.** Shari will eat, bathe, brush her teeth, and care for her hair, within 2 weeks (Insert date)	**a.** Will eat with assistance on the unit for 5 days (Insert date) Will bathe, brush teeth, and comb hair with supervision and assistance, as needed, daily for 1 week (Insert date)	Sit with Shari while she's eating. Encourage and feed, as necessary. Plan for supplemental snacks. Supervise and assist Shari, as needed, in daily bathing, oral hygiene, and hair care.
			b. Will eat in the dining room with other clients, within 1 week (Insert date). Will bathe, brush teeth, and comb her hair independently, within 12 days (Insert date)	Encourage Shari to make decisions and assume responsibility for her personal care. Praise her when she does things for herself and let her know that she can trust herself to make choices. (Increase self esteem.)

OVERLY SUSPICIOUS PATTERN OF BEHAVIOR

DESCRIPTION

The overly suspicious pattern of behavior is usually seen in people suffering from a paranoid disorder. These clients have usually had a childhood in which distrust, hate, and poor interpersonal relationships developed. As a result, severe feelings of inadequacy and inferiority interfere with the client's ability to look at and accept his own shortcomings. He denies the shortcomings to himself and uses the coping/mental mechanism of *projection* to attribute his feelings to objects and people outside himself. In doing so, the client feels more comfortable with himself and superior to others. He is a lonely person, frightened of being exposed as inadequate. As his anxiety increases, he manifests ideas of persecution. Statements such as, "You don't like me" reflect the projective technique. In reality, the client is saying he does not trust himself. His ideas are fixed and cannot be changed because his behavior is an attempt to meet a basic need to feel significant. Until he finds a more constructive way to meet this need, he will not give up his distorted ideas.

INTERVENTIONS

Caring for the overly suspicious client is challenging, easier to plan than to do. The client sets up obstacles for care through attitudes of superiority, ridicule, and sarcasm. He is inflexible and afraid of change. The client irritates and arouses aggressive feelings in others. Consequently, the health provider must deal with his own feelings before he can deal with the client nondefensively. Tact and courtesy are necessary in dealing with the client's negative behavior and emotions. Ridicule and sarcasm from the client must never be met with retaliation. For example, never speak sharply to the client or make fun of his ideas. Listen to the client's story, but neither agree nor disagree. Respond to the client's direct questions about his ideas calmly and matter-of-factly. The exact words will vary with the health provider, but two ideas to be conveyed are (1) understanding and (2) reality. A suggested response might be, "I know this is real to you, but I do not see it that way and it is not reality." Rudden, Gilmore, and Francis (1982) suggest that "confrontation with reality may have an important role in the evaluation and treatment of delusional patients." Whenever possible, praise the client for accomplishments. Sometimes allowing the client to assist with the care of a helpless client will enhance his feeling of importance. Give honest, specific praise rather than overall compliments. For example, say, "Thank you for walking up and down the hall with John," rather than, "You did a great job with John."

The health provider must be professional at all times and sensitive to the client's need for space. In addition, he must proceed slowly, taking cues from the client. The client is best approached on a one-to-one basis. He does not function well in groups or in competitive situations. The suspicious client often identifies others' behavior as referring to him (ideas of reference). Whispering or telling secrets may arouse further suspicion. Before he can learn to trust another person, he must learn to trust himself. In a one-to-one relationship, the health provider can help by identifying the times that trust occurs in the client's behavior. For example, when the client makes a positive decision about his life, the health provider can respond by saying, "That was a positive choice you made. See, you can trust your decisions."

Being honest with the client is essential. Frequently, the client will give the health provider clues as to when a sense of trust has been established by allowing the health provider into his space. He will then begin to test reality and make demands on the environment. For example, if the client thinks his food is poisoned, it may be necessary to serve food in closed containers and to allow the client to open the containers. Sometimes the client may want you to taste his food before he will eat it. Before tasting it, ask him which utensil he wants you to use and which part of the food he wants you to taste.

The overly suspicious client is always potentially dangerous to himself and others. He will need constructive outlets for his anger and aggressive drives. Tuning in to early behavior clues (e.g., angry facial expression, flushed face, tremulous voice, limited attention span), and actively intervening will prevent later violent outbursts. Noncompetitive solitary tasks, such as puzzles, ceramics, punching bag, or running, are therapeutic. All require some concentration, yet do not require the client to compete or cooperate with others.

As the client finds alternatives for dealing with his strong feelings and develops trust in himself and his environment, he begins to move into group activities. Once the client experiences success in group relations, he is well on his way to a healthier state of being.

The Essential Components of a Plan of Care for a Client with an Overly Suspicious Pattern of Behavior

Mr. Henry Heigel is 40 years old, about six feet tall, and has black hair. He is a lawyer who constantly quotes legal statutes that personnel have supposedly violated while giving him care. He insists that the bank owes him $50,000, which it doesn't, and he wants to leave the hospital to get the money. He feels superior to the other clients and refuses all medication because he feels the staff are trying to change him. He is well-informed on current events.

THE ESSENTIAL COMPONENTS OF A PLAN OF CARE FOR A CLIENT WITH AN OVERLY SUSPICIOUS PATTERN OF BEHAVIOR

STRENGTHS: Well educated, informed on current events   **Revision Date:** Insert date

DATE	NEED/PROBLEM	GOALS		APPROACH
		LONG-TERM GOALS (LTG)	**SHORT-TERM GOALS (STG)**	
Insert date	**1.** Inability to trust, as evidenced by delusion about bank owing him money and staff trying to change him with medication.	**1.** Mr. Heigle will develop trust in others by verbalizing that he no longer believes that the bank owes him money and that the staff are trying to change him through medication, within 3 weeks (Insert date)	**a.** Will take medication orally or by injection, within 3 days (Insert date)	Use client's proper name and title (i.e., Mr. Heigel) when requesting him to take medication. Offer medication orally; if he refuses, calmly state that it will be given to him intramuscularly, since his medications are court ordered. (Nonpunitive attitude is essential; be professional at all times.)
			b. Will limit his delusional verbalizations to sessions with his case manager twice daily, within 1 week (Insert date)	Do not argue or disagree with client's delusional ideas. Remind him that he is to speak of these to his case manager only. (His ideas are fixed.)
			c. Will write a feature article for the hospital newspaper, within 2½ weeks (Insert date)	Praise client for his real ability and accomplishments. (Contributes to a realistic sense of importance and trust in self; provides outlet for aggressive drives.)

DEPRESSIVE PATTERN OF BEHAVIOR

Many theories exist as to why an individual becomes clinically depressed. Some of these include the inability to deal with angry feelings, causing anger to be turned in on oneself; learned helplessness—"It's no use, nothing will help;" the cognitive theory, which focuses on negative thinking; and the biological theory, which is based on the assumption that biochemical and genetic factors cause depression. Despite the reason, the basic behavior that presents itself in all clinical depression is that of low self-esteem.

DESCRIPTION

The client who is clinically depressed can deal with his anger through the coping technique of *introjection*. By turning his anger in on himself—intra-aggression—it no longer poses an external threat to him as an individual. However, the client feels guilty about his anger and verbalizes his feelings through self-depreciation. Such statements as "Why do you waste your time on me?" or "Why don't you talk to someone more deserving?" are repeated over and over. The client's entire conversation centers around himself, and his relationships are immature and dependent.

The appearance of the depressed client is also distinctive. His face appears deeply sad and hopeless; his posture is usually stooped; and all of his body movements are slow, even though he may pace back and forth. The pacing is a way of dealing with his anxiety and has previously been referred to as agitated depression.

INTERVENTIONS

The health provider feels his client's depression. The client's depression is obvious. The health provider must remember that this individual needs to feel this way at this time in order to deal with his guilt and ultimate anger. Therefore, it is useless to reassure the client that he is worthy, since he needs to feel unworthy.

The client's ability to process information is decreased. Sometimes just being with the client without trying to carry on a conversation is the most reassuring thing that you can do. For example, it may be helpful to tell the client, "You do not need to talk; I just want to sit with you for awhile." When you leave, tell him, "I'm leaving now. I'll be back before I leave work at 3:00 p.m."

All internal body functions are slowed down, so elimination, eating, and sleeping can become problems. The health provider must evaluate and provide for the client's physical care.

When depression is severe, it is important to keep the client's life simple and make minimum demands upon him. Menial tasks or hard work may be a way of dealing constructively with the client's covert anger or need for self-punishment. Asking the client to do something for himself is usually unsuccessful, since he feels unworthy; however, he might be receptive to doing something for you if it is a sincere request. For example, "I am pressed for time. I'd appreciate it if you would help me fold the laundry." Upon completing the task, thank him for his contribution. Don't overdo it; keep the "thank you" simple and task-related. If the client expresses his hostility outwardly in a positive way, this is a good sign. The health provider should use this opportunity to support the client, sharing with him the benefits of dealing with anger constructively. For example, "I am glad you told me you did not want to go outside with the group."

Early morning hours are difficult for the depressed client because he has had a disruptive sleep. When he awakes, he feels no better than he did before he went to bed. Usually there is a period in early evening when the depression lifts slightly. Use this time to reach the client and share simple activities with him.

The Essential Components of a Plan of Care for a Client with a Depressive Pattern of Behavior

Mrs. Motley is a 50-year-old, white-haired woman who moves very slowly about the unit. Her face is haggard-looking, and her head is bent low. She repeatedly states that she is unworthy to have any care and wonders why the nursing personnel bother with her. She says, "I wish I were dead." She neglects her personal appearance because she doesn't deserve to look nice. While her children were at home, she was very neat and meticulous about her housekeeping. At present her appetite is poor, and she insists that she doesn't sleep much at night.

THE ESSENTIAL COMPONENTS OF A PLAN OF CARE FOR A CLIENT WITH A DEPRESSIVE PATTERN OF BEHAVIOR

STRENGTHS: Housekeeping skills, physically active   **Revision Date: Insert date**

DATE	NEED/PROBLEM	GOALS		APPROACH
		LONG-TERM GOALS (LTG)	**SHORT-TERM GOALS (STG)**	
Insert date	**1.** Negative ideas about self, such as unworthiness, not deserving to	**1.** Mrs. Motley will stop criticizing herself, within 1 month (Insert date)	**a.** Will take medication as prescribed, within 2 days (Insert date)	Give medication as ordered. Monitor closely for side effects. Offer simple explanation to client on how soon

THE ESSENTIAL COMPONENTS OF A PLAN OF CARE FOR A CLIENT WITH A DEPRESSIVE PATTERN OF BEHAVIOR—*Continued*

STRENGTHS: Housekeeping skills, physically active

Revision Date: Insert date

DATE	NEED/PROBLEM	GOALS		APPROACH
		LONG-TERM GOALS (LTG)	**SHORT-TERM GOALS (STG)**	
	look nice, and wishing she were dead.			medication is expected to work and on side effects, if they occur. (Provides needed information and involves client in care.)
			b. Will accept health provider just sitting with her, upon admission (Insert date)	Sit with client. Avoid over-cheerfulness. Tell her that she does not have to respond. Let her know when you are going to leave and when you will return. Do not try to convince her that her ideas about herself are wrong. (Needs her symptoms at this time.)
			c. Will assist the health provider in a simple task on the unit, such as folding laundry, within 2 weeks (Insert date)	Tell Mrs. Motley that you want her to come and help you fold the clothes now. (Take positive approach.) Always express your appreciation for her help with the specific task. (Increase self-esteem.)
Insert date	**2.** Has neglected her physical needs, such as personal hygiene, eating, and sleep.	**2.** Mrs. Motley will care for her own personal hygiene, eat a regular diet, and sleep through the night, within 3 weeks (Insert date)	**a.** Will care for her personal needs with minimum supervision, within 2 weeks (Insert date). Will accept warm milk to sleep at night, within 2 weeks (Insert date)	Initially perform all personal care for Mrs. Motley; gradually withdraw assistance as she is able to care for herself. Offer positive reinforcement for what she accomplishes. (Meet physical needs.)
			b. Will care for personal needs with occasional reminders, within 2½ weeks (Insert date)	
			c. Will begin to eat a regular diet, within 2½ weeks (Insert date)	

OVERACTIVE (MANIC) PATTERN OF BEHAVIOR

DESCRIPTION

The client with overactive behavior uses the technique of *projection* to turn his anger outward toward objects and people in his environment. He vents his anger through outbursts of frantic activity, criticism, sarcasm, vulgarity, and resentment of authority. His frantic activity, which makes both emotional and physical care difficult, is an attempt to increase his self-esteem.

INTERVENTIONS

The client needs a nonchallenging atmosphere and health providers who can accept his verbal abuse calmly and matter-of-factly. Anything less tends to increase the client's guilt feelings. Limit-setting is also necessary. Set limits on behavior that is harmful to the client or others, as well as on behavior that interferes with others' rights. Ignore the client's attempts to belittle staff, as well as vulgar conversation and speech. The client needs protection from overstimulation. A quiet area removed from the center of activity is often helpful. The client has a poor attention span and so is easily distracted. Use this distractibility to avoid difficult situations whenever possible. In distracting the aggressive client, you will need to provide constructive outlets for his excessive energy, such as the punching bag, jogging, tearing rags, housekeeping tasks, and volleyball. Finger and brush painting are often a good medium for expressing anger. The client needs constant reassurance that he is a worthy human being.

The client's elevated mood and overactivity may appear humorous. However, take care not to encourage this type of behavior. Laugh *with* the client, but not *at* him. Frequently, you can detect the depression that is beneath the false gaiety. The health provider is responsible for preventing the client from humiliating himself in front of others.

The overactive client neglects his physical needs. He is too busy to eat, sleep, or tend to personal grooming. It is important to help the client with any or all of these needs until he is capable of meeting them himself. An overactive client is sometimes an asset with withdrawn or depressed clients. The overactive client may be able to stimulate activity, even though his own distractibility will not permit him to follow through. Since the overactive client has difficulty completing his responsibilities, the health provider must control the number of functions he assumes.

The Essential Components of a Plan of Care for a Client with an Overactive (Manic) Pattern of Behavior

Mr. Rally is a 45-year-old salesman who is rather short and bald. He appears to be always going somewhere or doing something when on the unit. He continually interrupts conversations among staff, and if staff members do not focus on him at the time, he pokes them. He is very critical of how the unit is run and tries to make staff feel inadequate. He has big ideas for making money, but they never work out. He eats hurriedly and is too busy to care for his personal needs.

THE ESSENTIAL COMPONENTS OF A PLAN OF CARE FOR A CLIENT WITH AN OVERACTIVE (MANIC) PATTERN OF BEHAVIOR

STRENGTHS: Salesman's skills, big ideas, initiates contact, physically active

Revision Date: Insert date

DATE	NEED/PROBLEM	GOALS		APPROACH
		LONG-TERM GOALS (LTG)	**SHORT-TERM GOALS (STG)**	
Insert date	**1.** Increased physical and verbal activity manifested by constant motion and continual interruption of staff.	**1.** Mr. Rally will channel his energy constructively through an industrial assignment, within 2½ weeks (Insert date)	**a.** Will take prescribed medication, within 3 days (Insert date)	Give medication and monitor blood level, as ordered. Teach client relation of medication to illness when client is ready. (Will encourage compliance with treatment.)
			b. Will contact only his assigned health provider for his requests,	Maintain a calm, matter-of-fact manner when client pokes you or is sarcastic and

THE ESSENTIAL COMPONENTS OF A PLAN OF CARE FOR A CLIENT WITH AN OVERACTIVE (MANIC) PATTERN OF BEHAVIOR—*Continued*

STRENGTHS: Salesman's skills, big ideas, initiates contact, physically active

Revision Date: Insert date

DATE	NEED/PROBLEM	GOALS		APPROACH
		LONG-TERM GOALS (LTG)	**SHORT-TERM GOALS (STG)**	
			within 10 days (Insert date)	critical of you and the unit. Do not take such remarks personally. Refer him to his assigned health provider for his requests. (Take non-defensive approach.)
			c. Will work with health provider to clean his room, within 7 days (Insert date)	Distract client when he is over-active. Get him to clean his room or involve him in some similar activity that he can complete in a short time. His attention span is short, so change activities frequently. (Channel energies.)
Insert date	**2.** Too busy to eat and care for his personal needs.	**2.** Mr. Rally will sit down, eat a regular meal in the dining room, and take care of his personal hygiene, within 7 days (Insert date)	**a.** Will eat by himself in his own room with supervision, within 3 days (Insert date)	Offer finger foods and high-calorie liquids. Remove him to nonstimulating area, such as his room, and stay with him. (Meet nutritional needs.)
			b. Will accept assistance with his physical care and in selection of wearing apparel, within 5 days (Insert date)	Remind client to go to the toilet, to brush his teeth, and to bathe. With his assistance, select comfortable and neat appearing clothing for him. (Meet physical needs.)

SUICIDAL PATTERN OF BEHAVIOR

DESCRIPTION

Suicide is the deliberate ending of one's own life. Many myths or misconceptions have developed about suicide, including (Horoshak, 1977: 62).

MYTH	FACT
1. Persons who talk about suicide don't commit it.	1. In reality, four fifths of those who talk about suicide end up killing themselves.
2. Suicide happens without warning.	2. Although it may seem sudden, many clues and warnings—frequently referred to as a "cry for help"—are given.
3. Suicidal persons are determined to kill themselves.	3. The desire to live is part of the human condition. Persons contemplating suicide are struggling with

ambivalent desires to live and to die. The basic wish to live provides a key for intervention. Persons who have attempted suicide and have recovered frequently say that suicide seemed like the only way to relieve their intense emotional pain.

4. Improvement following a suicide attempt means the suicide risk is gone.

4. The most dangerous time for suicide is during the convalescent period and shortly after the individual starts taking antidepressants, since during these times the individual has more energy to put his self-destructive thoughts into action.

5. Persons who commit suicide are mentally ill.

5. Many times the actual suicide act is an impulsive one, resulting from extreme unhappiness or anger, especially among the younger population.

6. It is not a suicide unless there is a suicide note.

6. Only a small percentage of those who actually commit suicide leaves notes. Many of the deaths that are listed as accidents, such as one-car incidents, are actually suicides.

Although suicide has become the second cause of death among youth between the ages of 15 and 24 years (accidents are first), the elderly continue to have the highest number of suicides (Husain, Vandiver, 1984: 97). Depression has always increased the risk of suicide, as well as crisis situations, disease, and drugs and alcohol.

The health provider must be alert to possible clues of an impending suicide. Some of these clues include previous suicide attempts; threats; extreme depression, which includes sadness and lack of interest in work or friends; personality changes (e.g., sleeplessness, loss of appetite / weight, tendency to withdraw); preparations for death (e.g., putting affairs in order, giving away prized possessions—especially among the young); acquiring the means to commit suicide; a sudden lift in spirits that can mean the person is relieved because his problems will soon be over—"the calm before the storm."

INTERVENTIONS

The person who is contemplating suicide needs active emotional support. A significant other to whom the potential suicide victim can turn in time of need is essential. Some guidelines for interacting with the suicidal person follow (Frederick, 1976: 8–11):

1. Listen attentively; that is, try to understand the feeling behind the words.

2. Evaluate the seriousness of the individual's thoughts and feelings. If definite suicide plans have been made, consider the problem more acute than if the individual's suicidal thinking is vague.

3. Evaluate the intensity of the emotional disturbance. Agitation and restlessness in an individual who has been depressed are causes for alarm.

4. Take every complaint and feeling the individual expresses seriously. Do not undervalue what the person is saying.

5. Do not be afraid to ask directly if the individual has suicidal thoughts. Talking about it frankly can help prevent an individual from carrying out his idea. He usually welcomes the opportunity to open up and discuss it.

6. Don't be misled by comments that the individual is past his emotional crisis. Follow-up is important.

7. Be affirmative but supportive. Strong, definite guidelines are essential for a distressed individual. Provide emotional strength by communicating that you know what you are doing and that everything possible will be done for the individual.

8. Evaluate the individual's resources—his strengths, both internal and external. He

may have effective coping mechanisms that can be strengthened, and persons in his environment, such as a minister, relatives, and friends, who can be contacted.

9. Act specifically. Give the individual an assignment, such as the No-Decision Suicide Contract (Drye 1973:172). Under the contract, the individual agrees not to *accidentally* or *purposely* do anything to himself for _____ (put in time period). It is important to stress the accidental aspect of the agreement.

10. Do not avoid asking for assistance and consultation. Call upon whoever is needed, depending upon the severity of the case.

11. Make the environment as safe and unchallenging as possible. If necessary, maintain constant supervision during the suicide crisis.

12. Give reassurance that the individual's feelings of despair and pain are temporary and will pass. Encourage a change of pace, such as exercise or relaxation techniques. Avoid cliches, such as "Everything will be all right" and "Don't worry." These statements indicate a lack of sensitivity to the client's problem.

13. Mention that as long as life exists, there is a chance for help; but death is final.

14. Talk about the survivors who will become victims if the individual follows through with his self-destructive act. Remind him that if he is seeking revenge, he will not be around to enjoy the effects.

15. Never promise the individual that you will prevent him from committing suicide.

16. Do not challenge the individual in order to shock him out of his ideas. For example, never say, "You haven't the guts to do it." Also, arguing with the individual or analyzing his motives is useless. Never say, "You're just talking that way because you've had too much to drink," or "How can you think of suicide; you have so much to live for?"

If the individual succeeds in taking his life, the health provider should participate in a psychological autopsy at which he can share his feelings and receive support from his peers. The health provider must remember that if the individual commits suicide, despite intervention attempts, it was the individual's decision to end his life.

The Essential Components of a Plan of Care for a Client with a Suicidal Pattern of Behavior

Julia Delmar is an attractive woman in her late thirties who was admitted to the psychiatric unit after a suicide attempt from an overdose of Valium and alcohol. Her husband recently left her for another woman. She believes that he doesn't care if she lives or dies. Basically, she is a dependent person and has never been able to do anything on her own. Her friend, Patti, is her only close contact. She called her before she overdosed and asked her to look after her husband.

THE ESSENTIAL COMPONENTS OF A PLAN OF CARE FOR A CLIENT WITH A SUICIDAL PATTERN OF BEHAVIOR

STRENGTHS: Attractive; close friend, Patti

Revision Date: Insert date

DATE	NEED/PROBLEM	GOALS		APPROACH
		LONG-TERM GOALS (LTG)	SHORT-TERM GOALS (STG)	
Insert date	1. Attempted suicide with medication and alcohol.	1. Julia Delmar will find a positive solution to her present crisis, such as a job or training	a. Will begin to grieve the loss of her husband, within 1 week (Insert date)	Initiate acute suicidal precautions during admission. Encourage her to talk in detail about her suicide attempt and to contact her

Table continues on following page.

**THE ESSENTIAL COMPONENTS OF A PLAN OF CARE FOR A CLIENT WITH A
SUICIDAL PATTERN OF BEHAVIOR—*Continued***

STRENGTHS: Attractive; close friend, Patti
Revision Date: Insert date

DATE	NEED/PROBLEM	GOALS		APPROACH
		LONG-TERM GOALS (LTG)	**SHORT-TERM GOALS (STG)**	
		program that will lead to employment, within 3 weeks (Insert date)		close friend, Patti, for support. (Safety, security, and ventilation.) Give her permission to grieve the loss of her husband. (Important to mourn loss.)
			b. Will explore healthy alternatives, such as assertiveness training, to deal with her life crisis, within 2 weeks (Insert date)	Teach her the steps of the problem-solving process, and support her in applying these steps to her problem. (A way of exploring positive alternatives.) Refer her to vocational services for an industrial work placement in the hospital and for vocational counseling. (Identify positive future alternatives.)

BEHAVIOR PATTERNS OF THE YOUNG, CHRONICALLY MENTALLY ILL

DESCRIPTION

The young, chronically ill population is made up primarily of previously institutionalized clients. Many of these clients deny the need for treatment, fail to take their psychotherapeutic medications, and medicate themselves with street drugs. Two important factors seem to be involved: (1) the client views the admission of mental illness as being equal with failure, and (2) the natural rebelliousness of this age group. Among the young, rebellion is directed toward the mental health system, which represents authority.

Since today deinstitutionalization is emphasized, hospitalizations are brief. Consequently, many of these individuals drift from place to place. "Young chronics become drifters for many reasons: to leave problems and failures behind, to try to find or avoid closeness, to search for autonomy or avoid involvement in a treatment program" (Lamb, 1982:9). The older, over-30 age group does not move as much and are usually found in rooming homes, half-way houses, group homes, and nursing homes. They seem not to have the personal goals of the younger group and have given in to dependency upon the mental health system.

A small group of the young, chronically ill are involved in violent behavior directed toward others or themselves. "They often require highly structured community settings such as locked skilled nursing facilities or extended stays in state hospitals" (Lamb, 1982:9). Health providers are frequently involved with the young, chronically ill in the institutional setting as a result of the frequently repeated hospitalizations. The cycle of hospitalization—some improvement, community placement, lack of follow-through with therapy, decompensation, rehospitalization—continues. Because the client is often rebellious and provocative, health providers may tire of working with him and fail to give the client the care he deserves. The important work by health providers needs to be done before *regression* becomes fixed.

INTERVENTIONS

1. Be realistic in regard to goals. Mainstreaming this patient is usually unsuccessful, but improving his quality of life is realistic (Lamb, 1982:9). This can be done by:

   a. Interesting him in something outside himself, such as projects, other people, structured activities.

   b. Developing interest in sheltered employment or entry level jobs.

   c. Encouraging involvement with a support system. Depending on availability and the client's needs, the support system can include any of the following:

   (1) *Stable one-to-one* therapeutic relationship

   (2) *Co-therapeutic* relationships. This may prevent the client from feeling abandoned when one therapist is not available.

   (3) *Group therapy.* "Dependency needs can often be more usefully met over a long period of time with a group approach" (Pyke, 1982:83).

   (4) *Follow-up home visits.* An after-care program for chronically mentally ill clients may be available. If so, the client should meet the after-care worker prior to discharge.

   (5) *Involvement in social therapeutic* groups in the community, if available.

2. Help the client develop *rationalization* for why he may not be ready to take on too large a task, such as a difficult job or a demanding collegiate program. Failure would further deflate his ego and evoke guilt about having failed you after all you did for him.

3. Make changes slowly. For example, any change in therapy, such as a new therapist, a therapist's vacation, or community placement, must be dealt with in advance.

4. The health provider's attitude is important. Remember that although the client is chronically ill, he is responding to the age-related needs of his age group. Becoming angry with him because he does not succeed as readily as we desire only increases his problems.

The Essential Components of a Plan of Care for a Young, Chronically Ill Client

Shelley Talish is a 26-year-old client with a history of repeated psychotic episodes and multiple hospitalization since age 17. She also has a history of violent physical and verbal outbursts that have led to her removal from several half-way house and foster home placements. Her parents refuse contact with her. Her recent return from conditional release was prompted by a physical outburst directed at the houseparent at her last half-way house. When she secluded herself in her room, the houseparent called the police. When entry was finally made into the room, Shelley was found to have made multiple superficial cuts on her left forearm. "They said I was bad," she commented, looking off in another direction.

When Shelley arrived at the center, she seemed tense and frightened. Physically, she appeared tiny and helpless. It was difficult to imagine that she had blackened the houseparent's eye. Shelley's after-care worker was contacted and was present during the interview. According to the after-care worker, Shelley became angry when the houseparent told her to make her bed and clean her room. Shelley had stopped taking her medication several weeks before the incident. According to Shelley, "It made me feel better not to take my pills." She had been working five hours a day at the sheltered workshop, until three days ago, when she refused to go to work even after she had been encouraged to do so. Further questioning revealed that lately she had been hearing voices again, voices that told her she was bad and needed to be hurt.

THE ESSENTIAL COMPONENTS OF A PLAN OF CARE FOR A YOUNG CLIENT WITH CHRONIC MENTAL ILLNESS

STRENGTHS: Young, has lived outside the treatment facility, recently involved with sheltered workshop

Revision Date: Insert date

DATE	NEED/PROBLEM	GOALS		APPROACH
		ACTIVE GOALS	MAINTENANCE GOALS	
Insert date	1. Temporary problem (T.P.): Alteration in skin integrity of left forearm related to self cutting—superficial.	1. Open areas will decrease in size and heal without complication. Evaluate in 5 days (Insert date)		Observe and record condition of cuts on left forearm once each shift. Instruct and supervise Shelley's washing of left forearm with soap and water on day and evening shift. (Take care of physical needs.)
Insert date	2. Alteration in perception related to exacerbation of psychotic symptoms, evidenced by physical acting out toward houseparent and auditory hallucinations that tell her she is bad.	2a. Shelley will monitor situations that lead to physical outbursts, within 3 weeks (Insert date)		Administer medication as ordered. Shelley will go to her room for 10 minutes when she feels like striking out or until she feels in control (maximum 20 minutes). Staff may cue Shelley with, "Shelley, room." Staff will escort Shelley to her room for striking out. Shelley will stay there for 20 minutes or until she feels in control (maximum 30 minutes). Shelley will earn a 3-hour pass when she has successfully controlled her behavior on 3 successive days by going to her room. (Teaches a personal way to control behavior.)
		2b. Shelley will dismiss the "voices" herself, within 2 weeks (Insert date), beginning in 1 week (Insert date)		Shelley will be assigned to the same staff persons whenever possible. Morning and evening staff will contact Shelley 4 times per shift for 10 minutes. Night staff will contact Shelley in same way if she is awake. Staff will not ask for details regarding voices.

THE ESSENTIAL COMPONENTS OF A PLAN OF CARE FOR A
YOUNG CLIENT WITH CHRONIC MENTAL ILLNESS—*Continued*

| STRENGTHS: | Young, has lived outside the treatment facility, recently involved with sheltered workshop | | | Revision Date: | Insert date |

DATE	NEED/PROBLEM	GOALS		APPROACH
		ACTIVE GOALS	**MAINTENANCE GOALS**	
				Staff will direct Shelley to tell the voices to "Go away" or to say, "I won't do what you tell me." This is anxiety producing; be prepared to reassure her.
				Prompt staff not assigned to Shelley to make short, positive contacts with her. (Increase own sense of control over symptoms.)
				Shelley may go to the canteen alone on any day she is free of voices. (Reinforcement.)
Insert date	**3.** Lack of continuity in functioning in the community as evidenced by repeated admissions and refusal by some facilities to take Shelley back.		**3a.** Shelley will maintain contact with the after-care worker throughout her hospitalization.	After-care workers will continue to visit Shelley weekly throughout her hospitalization, beginning with admission. (Continue ongoing support relationship; discharge planning.)
		3b. Shelley will contact sheltered workshop and request to return to her old job, within 3 weeks (Insert date)		Staff will remind Shelley to contact sheltered workshop for return to work.
			3c. Shelley will take her psychotherapeutic medication as ordered.	The medication nurse will discuss the importance of taking psychotherapeutic medication regularly and ways to cope with side effects. Will also discuss the possible use of an intramuscular, long-acting medication as an alternative, as per doctor's order, in 3 weeks. (Reinforce the use of court-ordered medications.)

7

SPECIFIC PATTERNS OF BEHAVIOR RELATED TO THE MINOR MENTAL DISORDERS AND PERSONALITY DISORDERS

LEARNING OBJECTIVES—Upon completing this chapter, the reader will be able to:

1. Give two identifying characteristics for the anxious pattern of behavior and the acting-out pattern of behavior.

2. List two significant interventions for the anxious pattern of behavior and the acting-out pattern of behavior.

ANXIOUS PATTERN OF BEHAVIOR

DESCRIPTION

Mild anxiety is a normal and often helpful emotion that alerts us to anticipated danger. It often occurs when a person is facing a new situation, such as a new job or task. The anxiety keys up the person's mind and body so that he is ready to give his best performance. It is important for a person to be aware of the anxiety and its cause. In this way, the person can use the anxiety to his advantage and utilize the problem-solving process to move through his anxiety in a constructive way. This experience helps develop the individual's personality and character.

Persons with overwhelming anxiety have failed to deal with their anxiety. They are still struggling to fulfill very basic needs of feeling secure, adequate, and independent. In an effort to protect themselves against repeated frustrations and failure, they begin to use certain coping techniques.

Through *repression*, they attempt to keep the threatening experiences and thoughts hidden. However, they expend so much energy in doing this that the coping/mental mechanism eventually fails. In an attempt to maintain their equilibrium and maintain contact with their environment, these individuals try other means of coping with their discomfort, which ultimately can interfere with their daily living activities.

Some of the coping techniques utilized include *denial, conversion, displacement, compensation, depression, fantasy,* and *anger.* These techniques can cause an individual to display extreme behaviors, such as exaggeration of normal fears (phobic disorder), repetitive thoughts or actions, despite the individual's awareness of the senselessness of the behavior (obsessive/compulsive disorder), and overwhelming feelings of apprehension accompanied by physical symptoms, such as dizziness, dyspnea, palpitations, chest pain, smothering sensation, hot and cold flashes, and shaking (panic disorder).

INTERVENTIONS

Helping anxious persons deal constructively with anxiety is the health provider's goal. Unless the health provider has recognized and evaluated his own responses to anxiety, he can unknowingly support the person's negative ways of attempting to cope with anxiety.

The most important quality for the health provider who is working with an anxious client is an attitude of acceptance. It is important for the health provider to remember that the client has the right to be as sick as he needs to be at this time. The issue is not whether the health provider approves of the client's behavior, but that the provider accepts and realizes that, at this time, this is the best the client can do.

The health provider relieves anxiety through his concern and respect for the client and through his skill in working with him. The provider's willingness to spend time with the client is more effective than an empty reassurance, such as, "Everything will be O.K." It is important for the health provider to evaluate what the client can and cannot do for himself. In areas of care where the client needs help, such as personal grooming, the health provider must use direct assistance.

In caring for the client with overwhelming anxiety, the focus of attention must be on the client and not on the symptoms. This means that every opportunity should be made to interact with the client when he is not talking about his symptoms. Therefore, when the client verbalizes many physical complaints, the health provider should listen and make a mental note for possible physical evaluation. He should not comment about the client's symptoms or inquire about how he feels. Rather, the health provider should communicate an understanding of how the client might be feeling inside by making a comment such as, "You seem anxious this morning, so I'll be with you for short periods throughout the day."

The Essential Components of a Plan of Care for a Client with Overwhelming Anxiety

Mrs. Hattie Golden is a 42-year-old married woman who paces the floor and talks continuously about her physical symptoms, such as difficult breathing, the pounding of her heart, sweating, and smothering sensations. She talks about a fear of dying and possibly going crazy. She says she feels insecure and inadequate, and she is indecisive. She was active in the local garden club and is known for her collection of African violets. During her hospitalization, she has neglected her personal hygiene and appearance.

THE ESSENTIAL COMPONENTS OF A PLAN OF CARE FOR A CLIENT WITH OVERWHELMING ANXIETY

STRENGTHS: Interest in gardening, especially African violets

Revision Date: Insert date

DATE	NEED/PROBLEM	GOALS		APPROACH
		LONG-TERM GOALS (LTG)	**SHORT-TERM GOALS (STG)**	
Insert date	1. Preoccupation with physical symptoms.	1. Ms. Golden will show interest outside of self by taking care of the African violets on the unit, within 1 month (Insert date)	a. Will observe health provider's care of African violets on unit for 1 week (Insert date)	Listen to Ms. Golden's complaints. Do not tell her that they are not real. (This is her way of coping with anxiety at this time.)

Table continues on following page.

THE ESSENTIAL COMPONENTS OF A PLAN OF CARE FOR A CLIENT WITH OVERWHELMING ANXIETY—*Continued*

STRENGTHS: Interest in gardening, especially African violets

Revision Date: Insert date

DATE	NEED/PROBLEM	GOALS		APPROACH
		LONG-TERM GOALS (LTG)	**SHORT-TERM GOALS (STG)**	
			b. Will care for the African violets with health provider's assistance for the next 2 weeks (Insert date)	Try to interest her in things outside herself. (You are accepting her and at the same time diverting her attention from herself.) Provide simple activities, such as care of plants on unit, that are within Ms. Golden's ability and at which she can succeed. (Attempts to increase self-esteem.)
Insert date	**2.** Neglect of personal hygiene and appearance.	**2.** Ms. Golden will take care of her personal needs, such as bathing, oral hygiene, hair care, and clothing, within 1 month (Insert date)	**a.** Will bathe, clean teeth, comb hair, and change clothing for 2 weeks with health provider's assistance (Insert date)	Provide Ms. Golden with towels, toothbrush and paste, comb and brush. Take her through the steps of brushing teeth and bathing. Limit choice of clothing apparel to two. (Decision making must be simple due to preoccupation and slow thought processes.)
			b. Will bathe, clean teeth, care for hair, and change clothing daily with direction from health provider, as needed, for 2 weeks (Insert date)	

ACTING-OUT PATTERN OF BEHAVIOR

DESCRIPTION

Adjustment to the demands of society varies from limited adjustment, as seen with the chronically mentally ill (CMI) client, to healthy adjustment. According to mental health statistics, a large segment of the population fits into the category of unhealthy adjustment, as evidenced by the negative feelings and actions they project against society. A common diagnosis for individuals who exhibit acting-out patterns of behavior is *antisocial personality disorder*. These individuals appear to operate on the pleasure principle, as though their consciences were not operating. The kind of behavior they engage in varies but is most commonly associated with areas in which strong values are usually held, such as aggressiveness and sexual impulses.

The acting-out pattern of behavior begins early in life. The adult is remembered as the child who "never did mind, regardless of the tears and promises." In adolescence, patterns of truancy, casual sexual relationships, drug and alcohol abuse, fights, stealing, and vandalism were common. From early on, the individual usually has had repeated bouts with the law, despite his promises not to repeat the offenses. He feels no real remorse for his actions and may explain a brutal act with a statement such as, "I just wanted to see what it felt like to cut the dog in half." Unlike other people involved with the law, this individual engages in a variety of criminal activities that frequently includes rape. The personality of the acting-out client is usually superficially charming, and he is quick to play one staff member against another. Occasionally, the client can persuade a new health provider to believe that he is the only one who has ever understood or listened. According to the client, all he needs is a chance, some money, a place to stay, and some help finding a job. Unfortunately, the health provider complies, only to find out too late that an additional characteristic of this individual includes pathological lying.

This individual may be seen in a mental health setting for a variety of reasons. He may be experiencing a superimposed psychosis; he may have abused alcohol or drugs or the courts may have sent him there for evaluation or to give him an opportunity to work on his underlying problems. His chances for making a healthy adjustment are guarded because he continues to engage in the behavior. Studies indicate that some of these individuals finally begin to "burn out" around age 40 and, consequently, settle into more socially acceptable behavior.

INTERVENTIONS

1. A thorough *orientation* to rules, regulations, and expectations of the environment is necessary.

2. The health provider's *attitude* is important. You will need to be firm, yet respectful. Remember that the client's behavior represents his defense against anxiety. He deals with his anxiety by immediately discharging it onto the environment in many destructive ways. He is sometimes referred to as an "actor on the stage of life."

3. Involve the client in a discussion about what is to be accomplished during his hospitalization.

4. Develop a structured plan for the day's activities. Review the plan with the client, being sure he understands it, and give him a copy of the plan.

5. Make *no* exceptions to the plan once it is instituted.

6. Have the client limit all of his requests to his assigned care-giver on each shift. Be sure that all staff are aware of the plan.

7. Record compliance with the plan on each shift. Remember that the client is entitled to honest feedback on how he is progressing.

8. When the individual begins to use his negative techniques, interrupt the behavior and point out what he is doing.

9. Know where the client is at all times. He may seek out clients with like problems or defenseless clients (e.g., the withdrawn client) to exploit them.

10. If the client has superimposed problems, such as psychosis or substance abuse, the specific additional interventions will have to be incorporated in his care.

The Essential Components of a Plan of Care for a Client with an Acting-Out Pattern of Behavior

Fred Markers, age 19, was admitted to the mental health center. He had been on the children's unit for 6 weeks at the age of 13. Fred has a history of numerous problems such as truancy from school, lying, running away from home, using drugs and alcohol, and frequent fights. Because of drug use and stealing, he appeared in juvenile court at age 15 but was dismissed for lack of evidence. This is the first time Mr. Markers has been in adult court for selling drugs. The judge listened to Mr. Markers' plea for a chance to "straighten out" and sent him to the mental health center for two weeks of observation. Mr. Markers is a tall, good-looking, charming young man who quickly involved himself in unit activities.

Later in the week, 3 clients reported missing money. Although the money was located in Mr. Markers' room, he denied taking it, adding, "Somebody planted it there. Another bum rap!" Later in the day, he sought out a new staff nurse. He talked to her about needing someone to understand him and give him a chance. He told her she was the first one who had ever really listened to him.

THE ESSENTIAL COMPONENTS OF A PLAN OF CARE FOR A CLIENT WITH AN ACTING OUT PATTERN OF BEHAVIOR

STRENGTHS: **Good looking, charming, young**   **Revision Date:** **Insert date**

DATE	NEED/PROBLEM	GOALS		APPROACH
		ACTIVE GOAL	**MAINTENANCE GOAL**	
Insert date	**1.** Socially unacceptable behavior that culminated in his arrest for selling drugs (Court observation)	**1.** Mr. Markers will behave in a socially acceptable manner while on the unit for observation for 2 weeks (Insert date)		Provide Mr. Markers with a thorough orientation to unit rules, regulations, and expectations. Give him a copy of the unit orientation booklet to refer to. (Identify expectations.) Instruct Mr. Markers to limit all of his requests on each shift to the staff person assigned to him. Make no exceptions to the rules. (Define limits.) Know where Mr. Markers is at all times, since he is under court observation. Do not allow passes or independent activities during the 2 week observation period. Police department has requested that they be notified should he leave. (Standard procedure per court.) Deal with all attempts at manipulation by interrupting the cycle and explaining to Mr. Markers what he is doing. (Decrease manipulation.) Note and carefully record Mr. Markers' behavior on each shift. (Required for court observation.) Instruct all staff to read and follow Mr. Markers' care plan. (Provide continuity and consistency.)

SPECIFIC PATTERNS OF BEHAVIOR RELATED TO CHILDHOOD DISORDERS

LEARNING OBJECTIVES—Upon completing this chapter, the reader will be able to:

1. Give two identifying characteristics for children with an emotionally disturbed pattern of behavior and a behavior pattern related to mental retardation with emotional disturbances.

2. List two significant interventions for children with an emotionally disturbed pattern of behavior and a behavior pattern related to mental retardation with emotional disturbances.

CHILDREN WITH AN EMOTIONALLY DISTURBED PATTERN OF BEHAVIOR

DESCRIPTION

The classes of this disorder, which are usually first evident in infancy, childhood, or adolescence, are separated into five major groups according to DSM-III (APA, 1980:35–36):

MAJOR GROUP	EXAMPLE OF DISORDER
1. Intellectual	Mental retardation
2. Behavioral	Attention deficit disorder
3. Emotional	Anxiety disorders of infancy, childhood, and adolescence
4. Physical	Eating disorders
5. Developmental	Pervasive development disorders

The major group designation identifies the predominant area of disturbance that prevents the child from coping successfully on the outside without mental health intervention.

In order to understand children with emotionally disturbed patterns of behavior and plan for their care, it is essential to have a good working knowledge of growth and development. Basically, growth and development are influenced by hereditary factors and environmental influences. These factors can work in either direction for the child. For example, he may have been able to compensate for his limitations because of opportunity and a supportive environment. On the other hand, the child may have inherited a great deal genetically but never reached his full potential because of a lack of opportunity and support in his environment.

INTERVENTIONS

The planned interventions for the child with an emotionally disturbed pattern of behavior are based on an assessment of the child by a skilled practitioner with excellent knowledge about growth and development levels and the associated needs for each level. What stands out is that the child may be functioning at several different levels of growth and development at the same time. The depth of *regression* must be identified, and the needs of the level the child has regressed to must be clarified. The child may continue to function at his chronological level in certain areas. For example, an eight-year-old who has temper tantrums may be functioning at a preschool level in regard to his emotional development. However, intellectually he may be at his chronological age or above.

Some suggested interventions dependent upon the level of growth and development are:

1. *Communication.* This must occur at the child's level of comprehension. To be sure the child has understood your intended message, have him repeat what you told him.

2. *Limit-setting.* Use a direct statement rather than a question, which offers a choice. For example, say, "I know you are angry, but you cannot hit me," rather than, "Why did you hit me?" The statement should be followed with information on what he can do. For example, "You can hit the punching bag in your room." When the negative behavior has subsided, talk to the client about what has occurred.

3. *A structured plan.* Develop a structured plan for the child daily. The child's commitment to change is essential. Once he accepts responsibility for change, excuses are not acceptable. Go through the plan with the client, and give him a copy of the plan. The child should be positively reinforced for what he achieves. Focus on what he has done correctly.

The goal in working with children is to teach them responsibility for their behavior and for meeting their own needs, since ultimately no one else can do it for them.

The Essential Components of a Plan of Care for a Child with an Emotionally Disturbed Pattern of Behavior

Bill, eight years of age, was admitted to the children's unit of the local community mental health center. The reason: Bill required constant supervision to be kept from disrupting classroom activities. He was described as stubborn, defiant, and quarrelsome and was said to have a short attention span.

At home, Bill was constantly moving, running, jumping, rocking, or "fooling around" with something. He started many projects at one time without completing any of them. He made poor judgments, and was constantly wandering off by himself to do whatever he wished. Consequently, he also needed constant supervision at home. He disrupted any activity going on in the household, provoking his older siblings.

Bill is a nice-looking, friendly boy. He is agile and is constantly moving on the unit. He can be distracted easily. Bill has stated that he is "O.K." and doesn't have any fears.

THE ESSENTIAL COMPONENTS OF A PLAN OF CARE FOR AN EMOTIONALLY DISTURBED CHILD

STRENGTHS: Age, energy, nice looking, friendly, agile   **Revision Date:** Insert date

| DATE | NEED/PROBLEM | GOALS | | APPROACH |
		LONG-TERM GOALS (LTG)	SHORT-TERM GOALS (STG)	
Insert date	**1.** Involved in frantic, ceaseless activity that prevents him from functioning successfully at home and school.	**1.** Bill will show a reduction in anxiety, evidenced by a decrease in his motor activity on the unit, within 2 months (Insert date)	**a.** Will take prescribed medication on admission (Insert date)	Give medication as prescribed. Assign same health provider to work with him on each shift. (Develop a stable relationship.)
			b. Will focus on a single activity of his choice in a room by himself for 10 minutes twice daily, within one month (Insert date)	Provide a private room with minimum furnishings and nonstimulating colors. Offer only 2 games or activities, from which he will select one. (Decrease stimuli.) Praise him if he focuses on the activity for the specified time. (Positive reinforcement.)
Insert date	**2.** Stubborn, quarrelsome, defiant behavior interferes with his relationships with others.	**2.** Bill will show a decrease in his defiant behavior, as evidenced by his positive relationships with peers on the unit, within 2½ months (Insert date)	**a.** Will make his bed daily, by 1 month (Insert date)	Develop a structured plan at his level of functioning with built-in *positive reinforcers*, such as money for an ice cream cone at the canteen. (Increase self-esteem.)
			b. Will work with the health provider in cleaning up the playroom daily, by 1½ months (Insert date)	
			c. Will work with assigned peer to clean playroom, by 2 months (Insert date)	

BEHAVIOR PATTERN RELATED TO MENTAL RETARDATION AND EMOTIONAL DISTURBANCE

DESCRIPTION

To understand the special needs of the client who is mentally retarded and also emotionally disturbed, a review of some basic information about mental retardation is important. The definition of mental retardation offered by the American Association on Mental Deficiency is as follows: "Mental Retardation refers to significantly subaverage general intellectual functioning existing concurrently with deficits in adaptive behavior, and manifested during the developmental period." (Grossman, 1977:11) (This definition is in agreement with the definition of mental retardation provided by *DSM-III*, where it is listed under Intellectual Disorders in the section on "Infancy, Children or Adolescence Disorders.") Significantly *subaverage general intellectual functioning* is established at approximately 70 or below intelligence quotient (I.Q.). Normal I.Q. is approximately 100. *Deficit in adaptive behavior* refers to the inability to successfully learn the activities of daily living that help one cope independently on a day-to-day basis. The *developmental period* as identified in the DSM-III refers to an onset before age 18. The period includes prenatal development and the birth process.

Causes of retardation are usually biological or psychosocial or a combination of the two. The most common biological causes are Down's syndrome and phenylketonuria. Heavy alcohol consumption by the woman during pregnancy can result in fetal alcohol syndrome, which includes mental retardation. Psychosocial factors such as the lack of social and intellectual stimulation have also been shown to cause mental retardation. Dr. Marlin Roll's Pine School Project at the University of Iowa (late 1950's to early 1960's) identified a number of these children and showed that appropriate environmental stimulation could help many of them function at a higher level. If the stimulation was begun early enough during the preschool stage of development, many children functioned within a normal intelligence range. Malnutrition during infancy and childhood continues to produce mental retardation throughout the world. Often, many other abnormalities are associated with mental retardation. For example, neurological abnormalities such as seizures or problems with vision and hearing may be present. Mental disorders such as infantile autism and attention deficit disorders with hyperactivity are three to four times greater in children with mental retardation. Behavioral manifestations may occur, such as temper tantrums, aggressiveness, or irritability. For unknown reasons, more males than females develop mental retardation. The total population with mental retardation is about 1 per cent.

Mental retardation has four subtypes, each representing a particular amount of intellectual impairment:

Mild Mental Retardation.

This category represents about 80 percent of the mentally retarded population and is "roughly equivalent to the educational category 'educable'" (APA, 1980:39). During the preschool years, these persons can develop social and communication skills. By their late teens, they can learn academic skills of approximately a sixth grade level and often are not seen as different from other children until a later age. Many of them can learn vocational skills that will provide them with an opportunity to contribute to their own support. They continue to need guidance and support, especially during stressful times.

Moderate Mental Retardation.

According to DSM-III, this category makes up about 12 percent of the mentally retarded population and is roughly equivalent to what educators consider "trainable." These persons can learn simple language and speech, toilet training, and basic personal care. Academically, they progress to approximately a second grade level. Training in occupational skills is helpful, and many can, with supervision, assist in supporting themselves in sheltered workshop settings doing semiskilled or unskilled jobs. They benefit from additional supervision and guidance when under mild social or economic stress.

Severe Mental Retardation.

This group represents about 7 percent of the mentally retarded population. According to DSM-III, poor motor development and minimal speech is apparent during the preschool years. However, during the school-age period, some may learn to talk, and some may learn basic hygiene skills such as toilet training. Vocational training leading to simple work tasks under close supervision is possible.

Profound Mental Retardation.

This small group makes up approximately 1 percent of the mentally retarded population. Some may eventually be able to assist with self-care in a limited way. Constant aid and supervision will be necessary for the rest of their lives.

Sometimes mental retardation is confused with mental illness. They may exist together; however, mental retardation does not mean that a person is automatically mentally ill or vice versa. Table 8–1 points out some of the differences.

INTERVENTIONS

Adequate intervention in the care of the mentally retarded client with emotional problems is actually dual intervention that should be based on (1) the *degree of retardation* and (2) the *specific pattern of behavior* exhibited by the client.

The interventions that have been suggested for the various patterns of behavior form the basis for care. Modification in the approach depends on the retardation level. Therefore, an evaluation of the client's intellectual, social, physical, and behavioral functioning is essential as you prepare to individualize the care plan.

Some general interventions follow:

1. The client, although he may be an adult, acts and thinks like a child. It is important to meet the client at his level and proceed at his pace. However, in doing so, use adult materials. For example, if he is capable only of coloring, have the client color adult, rather than childish, pictures.

2. Establish an adult-to-adult relationship, rather than a parent-to-child relationship. Avoid using baby talk. Deliver messages simply, using the first person.

3. Because of his intellectual limitations, the mentally retarded client sometimes has difficulty understanding time spans. For example, telling the individual that his birthday is in two weeks is difficult for him to comprehend. Do not mention such events too far ahead of time.

4. Sometimes a mentally retarded client craves attention and will resort to any means to get it. In seeking the attention, he may become very possessive. The mentally retarded client should receive attention within limits, and the health provider, through a consistent approach, should adjust these limits as needed. Never provide attention one day and

TABLE 8–1. Comparison of Mental Illness and Mental Retardation

MENTAL ILLNESS	MENTAL RETARDATION
Mental illness is not directly related to intellectual functioning, although it may temporarily affect it.	Mental retardation refers to significantly subaverage general intellectual functioning.
Social adaptation depends on the severity of the mental illness.	The individual experiences a deficit in adaptive behavior (i.e., functions that help you make it through the day).
Mental illness can occur at any time in the life cycle.	Mental retardation occurs during the developmental period, with onset before age 18.
Mental illness is acute or chronic, depending on the type of illness. It may be functional or organic in nature.	Intellectual impairment is permanent but can be compensated for through development of the person's potential.
Socially inappropriate behavior often identifies the need for treatment.	The individual is expected to behave rationally for his level. He requires more support during mild stress. Prevalence of other disorders may create behavioral changes.

Data from *DSM-III*, pp. 36–40.

withdraw it the next day simply because you do not want to give it. Such inconsistency is hard for the mentally retarded client to understand.

5. Promises should not be made to the mentally retarded client unless they can be followed through.

6. The mentally retarded client should not be used to meet the health provider's needs, such as running errands or performing other tasks that are the health provider's responsibility.

7. Tolerance, a consistent approach, understanding, and supervision are most important in working with the mentally retarded client, with emphasis on normalization. Normalization means making available to the mentally retarded client patterns and conditions of everyday life that resemble, as closely as possible, the usual patterns of living for the average person in society. Strive constantly to develop whatever potential the client has. The more competent a person becomes, the more acceptable are his distortions.

The Essential Components of a Plan of Care for a Client Who Is Mentally Retarded and Emotionally Disturbed

Sally Dequaine is a 25-year-old short, obese, mentally retarded and emotionally disturbed woman who always has a grin on her face. She sits in a rocking chair most of the day holding a baby doll. Her speech is difficult to understand and consists mainly of single words. She is very aware of her surroundings and beams when a staff member spends some time with her; however, when she is out of her chair, she wanders into other clients' rooms and goes through their dresser drawers. She must be repeatedly reminded to comb her hair, brush her teeth, and take a bath. However, she is very willing to have staff do these things for her.

THE ESSENTIAL COMPONENTS OF A PLAN OF CARE FOR A CLIENT WITH MENTAL RETARDATION AND EMOTIONAL DISTURBANCE

STRENGTHS: Awareness of surroundings, pleasant disposition, can care for self with encouragement

Revision Date: Insert date

| DATE | NEED/PROBLEM | GOALS | | APPROACH |
		ACTIVE GOALS	MAINTENANCE GOALS	
Insert date	1. Decrease in intellectual functioning		1. Sally will maintain her present intellectual functioning.	Meet Sally at her level. Then proceed slowly at her pace. Remember that Sally thinks and acts like a child but chronologically is an adult. She needs kindness, patience, and interested staff to develop her potential. It is helpful if the same staff person works with Sally and extends to her the affection she needs. (Meeting client at her level of functioning.)
Insert date	2. Neglects personal care	2. Sally will brush her own teeth without being reminded, within 1 month (Insert date)		Break toothbrushing procedure into small steps, and use positive reinforcers, such as praise and spending time with her, after she accomplishes each step.

**THE ESSENTIAL COMPONENTS OF A PLAN OF CARE FOR A CLIENT WITH
MENTAL RETARDATION AND EMOTIONAL DISTURBANCE—*Continued***

| STRENGTHS: | Awareness of surroundings, pleasant disposition, can care for self with encouragement | | | Revision Date: | Insert date |

| DATE | NEED/PROBLEM | GOAL | | APPROACH |
		ACTIVE GOALS	MAINTENANCE GOALS	
				(Refer to Chapter on Applied Behavior Analysis for shaping.) Toothbrushing steps follow: —Pick up toothbrush and turn on water. —Wet brush under running water. —Squeeze toothpaste onto brush. —Brush back and forth on top of lower back teeth (both sides of mouth). —Brush back and forth under upper back teeth (both sides of mouth). —Brush down on all upper teeth. —Brush up on all lower teeth. —Rinse mouth. —Rinse toothbrush under running water. —Hang up brush.
Insert date	3. Wanders into other clients' rooms and goes through their dresser drawers	3. Sally will respond to cuing, "Sally, no," within 1 month (Insert date)		Provide ongoing close observation during each shift. Collect data on wandering, plus activity before and after wandering. Explain limit and cue to Sally. When she wanders, use the words, "Sally, no." When she responds to the cue, "Sally, no," immediately praise her.

SPECIFIC PATTERNS OF BEHAVIOR RELATED TO ORGANIC MENTAL DISORDERS

LEARNING OBJECTIVES—Upon completing this chapter, the reader will be able to:

1. Give two identifying characteristics for a behavior pattern related to organic changes in the brain and a behavior pattern related to the use of alcohol/drugs.

2. List two significant interventions for a behavior pattern related to organic changes in the brain and a behavior pattern related to the use of alcohol/drugs.

BEHAVIOR PATTERNS RELATED TO ORGANIC CHANGES IN THE BRAIN

DESCRIPTION

Oxygen, which is carried in the blood stream, is essential for brain functioning. When the brain is deprived of oxygen as a result of injury or disease, brain cells are damaged. Depending on the area of the brain and the number of cells involved, observable behavioral changes can occur. The behavioral changes are usually closely related to the individual's basic personality but are more exaggerated. Previously successful coping techniques are weakened as a result of the organic changes, allowing repressed emotional conflicts to surface.

Behavioral changes, according to *DSM-III* (APA, 1980:107–112), may include the following:

Memory Impairment. Memory impairment ranging from recent (forgetfulness in daily life, such as time and places) to remote (his own identity) occurs in severe organic disorders.

Impairment in Abstract Thinking. Accelerations or slowing of thought or total disorganization occur. The client cannot pull out significant parts of a statement and consequently interprets what is said concretely (literally). For example, he literally interprets the proverb, "A rolling stone gathers no moss," to mean that a stone in motion does not pick up anything, rather than as a reference to someone who moves frequently and never puts down roots.

Impaired Judgment and Impulse Control. Coarse language, inappropriate jokes, neglect of personal hygiene may be noted.

Other Higher Cortical Functions. Language changes, such as aphasia, mutism and failure to recognize objects, may develop.

Personality Change. This involves an alteration or exaggeration of premorbid traits, such as paranoia, compulsiveness, or irritability.

State of Consciousness. Clouding of consciousness can occur. The client may have difficulty engaging in conversation because his attention wanders.

Perceptual Disturbance. This can include misinterpretations (branch against the window misinterpreted as a burglar); illusions (lint on bedclothes seen as a bug); and hallucinations (most commonly visual, as in seeing something or someone who is not there).

Sleep-wakefulness Cycle. The cycle can range from simple drowsiness to stupor or semicoma. Or the client may have difficulty falling asleep. A reversed sleep-waking cycle can also occur, which usually involves vivid dreams or nightmares.

Psychomotor Activity. Changes vary from one extreme to another but usually involve restlessness or hyperactivity, groping or picking at bedclothes, attempts to get out of bed, striking out at objects that don't exist, sudden position changes, and decreased psychomotor activity from sluggishness to stupor.

Emotional Disturbances. Such disturbances may include fear, anxiety, depression, irritability, anger, euphoria or apathy (may vary or stay the same), or emotional lability (laughing or crying for no apparent reason).

Symptoms vary according to the type and extent of organic disorder the client experiences.

INTERVENTIONS

The health provider's most important attribute in regard to the organically impaired client is his attitude. Regardless of the extent of brain impairment, the client is a human being who is entitled to respectful and dignified care. "At the very least, you can attend carefully to your patients' physical needs. This way his mental dysfunction won't be aggravated by avoidable bodily deterioration or loss of self-image. More effective still, you can modify his environment so his disabilities aren't aggravated or allowed to overpower him. And finally, you can help him hold onto his human dignity by providing him with sensitive human interaction, even on a limited basis" (Richardson, 1982:67).

More specific care approaches for the organically impaired client include:

1. Establish a structured, consistent, daily routine.
2. Patiently answer questions in short, simple sentences. Repeat the answer as necessary.
3. Supervise health habits, including eating, personal hygiene, exercise, and toileting.
4. Have client assist with personal care as much as possible.
5. Demonstrate nonverbally and concretely what you are trying to convey to the client.
6. Tell the client when you do not understand what he is talking about.
7. Try to help the client, whenever necessary, become oriented through the use of clocks, calendars, signs, and written and verbal reminders.
8. Use the client's past memory to bring him to the present through reminiscing. For example, say, "You are in a nursing home now. But tell me about the time that you had a farm." In this way you are orienting the client to his present place while also allowing him to share with you his experiences of earlier years.
9. Be supportive of family members. The client is usually "not the person (we) used to know."

Caring for the client who is organically impaired presents a challenge. But the rewards from establishing a relationship with such a person cannot be measured.

The Essential Components of a Plan of Care for a Client with Organic Impairment of the Brain

Mr. Colter, age 80, is quite unsteady on his feet. At times he is disoriented in regard to time and place; his thoughts and conversations relate to the past, especially to his rock collection. He picks up small objects, such as buttons and chunks of bread and calls them rocks. He feels alone, unwanted, and helpless. He is impatient and tends to be bossy (like a parent). He dribbles urine and does not eat a balanced diet because his dentures do not fit well.

THE ESSENTIAL COMPONENTS OF A PLAN OF CARE FOR A CLIENT WITH ORGANIC BRAIN IMPAIRMENT

STRENGTHS: Rock collection, assertiveness   **Revision Date:** Insert date

DATE	NEED/PROBLEM	GOALS — ACTIVE GOALS	GOALS — MAINTENANCE GOALS	APPROACH
Insert date	**1.** Temporary problem (T.P.): Dentures do not fit well	**1.** Mr. Colter will see a dentist in 1 week for evaluation of his dentures (Insert date)		Have dentist check dentures. In meantime, contact dietitian regarding temporary change in diet. (Physical needs)
Insert date	**2.** Disoriented as to time and place	**2.** Mr. Colter will be able to repeat the time and place when it is reviewed with him daily.		Place a calendar and a clock with numbers in a convenient place. Orient Mr. Colter daily to month, day, time, and place. (Contact with reality)
Insert date	**3.** Is lonely, as evidenced by his bossiness	**3.** Mr. Colter will become involved with other clients on the unit by displaying his rock collection at the hobby show, in 2 weeks (Insert date)		Refer to Mr. Colter by title and last name, such as Mr. Colter, not Andy. Provide links with Mr. Colter's past (relatives or friends). Provide a small bag for his possessions (Hoarding). Show interest in what he carries around. Ask him to share with you some of his experiences. (Channel bossiness.) Provide consistent ward routine. Try not to move his bed, possessions, or place of eating. Write letters for Mr. Colter or offer the materials to him. Encourage him to make friends with other patients and to do as much as possible for himself. Use his special interests (his collection of rocks) to stimulate his participation in ward activities. (Make him feel a part of the group.)
Insert date	**4.** Unsteady on his feet		**4.** Mr. Colter will remain ambulatory as long as possible.	Assist Mr. Colter when he is walking. Do not use loose rugs; wipe up spills; have Mr. Colter wear shoes instead of slippers. (Safety)
Insert date	**5.** T.P.: Dribbling of urine	**5.** Mr. Colter will see the doctor for evaluation of his problem (Insert date)		Have doctor check Mr. Colter for dribbling of urine. In meantime, take Mr. Colter to the toilet at regular times, and be sure that his genital area is kept clean. Provide dry clothes as needed. (Personal hygiene)

BEHAVIOR PATTERN RELATED TO THE USE OF ALCOHOL/DRUGS

DESCRIPTION

Currently, the most abused drug in our society is alcohol. Although many people combine alcohol with other drugs or substances that are hazardous to the human body, this discussion will focus on alcohol abuse. Alcoholism has been viewed in many ways. In the nineteenth century, it was seen as a moral issue; the person who drank was a sinner. Today, some people still cling to this belief. Others view alcoholism as a disease, a learned behavior, a psychosocial condition, or a cultural trait. The common denominator in all cases of alcoholism is the serious physical and psychological reactions that occur with prolonged drinking. The World Health Organization defines alcoholism as follows:

> Alcoholics are those excessive drinkers whose dependence on alcohol has attained such a degree that it shows a noticeable mental disturbance or an interference with their bodily and mental health, their interpersonal relations and their smooth social and economic functioning, or who show the prodromal signs of such developments (WHO, 1951).

The physiological effects of alcohol consumption involve almost every organ in the body, including the mouth and throat, stomach, intestines, liver, pancreas, nerves, brain, heart, lung, and kidneys.

Psychologically, the alcoholic uses a myriad of coping/mental mechanisms, including *denial, projection, rationalization, repression,* and *suppression.* The alcoholic's use of denial perpetuates a continuous cycle of low self-concept, drinking to improve self-concept, guilt over behavior connected with drinking, and drinking again to deal with the guilty feelings. Other psychological factors that present problems include manipulation, dependency, depression and suicide, and loneliness (Estes et al., 1980:24–44).

INTERVENTION

Treatment for alcoholism/substance abuse involves three phases: detoxification, rehabilitation, and follow-up. Each stage is described below.

1. Detoxification. This is the period of abstinence from alcohol that follows a period of intoxication.
   a. Close observation of symptoms is necessary. According to *DSM-III* (APA, 1980:133–134), shortly after the reduction or discontinuation of alcohol ingestion, individuals in their thirties or forties who have been drinking since early in life may develop *alcohol withdrawal.* Major symptoms include coarse tremors of hands, tongue, and eyelids; nausea and vomiting; malaise or weakness; tachycardia; diaphoresis; hypertension; anxiety; depressed mood; irritability; and orthostatic hypotension. Grand mal seizures may also occur. Usually these symptoms disappear in five to seven days, unless *alcohol withdrawal delirium* develops. This syndrome, known also as *delirium tremens* (D.T.'s), may develop on the second or third day after drinking has stopped or been slowed down. Major symptoms are those of delirium (see Chapter 3), plus tachycardia, diaphoresis, and hypertension. Other symptoms that usually occur include delusions; vivid, visual hallucinations; and agitated behavior. The syndrome subsides in two to three days, unless complicated by another illness.
   b. Vital signs need to be monitored frequently to prevent complications.
   c. Maintain adequate hydration and nutritional intake with well-balanced meals and short-term vitamin therapy, if indicated.
   d. Provide a nonstimulating environment that is conducive to rest and relaxation. A quiet environment will eliminate unnecessary noises that can cause overreactions or seizures in the client. A well-lighted room will increase orientation and decrease hallucinations.

    e.   Note responses to questions and directions to determine level of consciousness.

    f.   Note changes in behavior in case it is necessary to implement medication therapy.

    g.   An accepting attitude on the part of the health provider is significant to the ultimate success or failure of treatment for the alcoholic client.

2.   Rehabilitation or Treatment. Rehabilitation for the alcoholic usually means a new life style—different friends, different job, different leisure activities. It means finding alternative ways of dealing with stress other than alcohol—ways that will produce "natural highs," such as running, meditating, and swimming.

    a.   Involve the client in developing his plan of care so that he assumes responsibility and accountability for his treatment.

    b.   Structure daily living and leisure time activities to provide consistency.

    c.   Set and maintain limits to minimize manipulative behavior.

    d.   Provide various group experiences, such as alcohol/drug education, Alcoholics Anonymous (A.A.) lessons and meetings, work opportunities, social interactions, family sessions, gripe sessions, values clarification sessions, relaxation techniques, nutritional groups, leisure counseling, job interviews, and community living skills.

3.   Follow-up Care. With the client, plan out-patient visits, individual counseling, group sessions, home/half-way house visits, and family counseling (Kreigh, Perko, 1983:379–380).

Regardless of the method used to treat the alcoholic, according to Michael Swift in his article, "How to Help an Alcoholic Who Insists He Doesn't Need Any Help," four steps are essential to any recovery:

1.   The alcoholic must accept the fact that he suffers from a chronic but treatable disease.

2.   He must stop drinking.

3.   He must be willing to do what is necessary to aid his recovery.

4.   He must come to accept life and himself for what they really are.

Essential Components of a Plan of Care for the Alcoholic Client

Mr. David Morgan, age 37, was brought to the chemical dependency unit by police. Neighbors had contacted the police upon observing Mr. Morgan almost hit a paperboy with his car after arriving home from a night of drinking. Mr. Morgan was accompanied by his wife, who was visibly upset and kept saying "Either shape up this time for good, or I'm leaving you. No more talking me into one more chance!" Mr. Morgan smelled heavily of alcohol and needed assistance from the car into the building. His speech was slurred, his face flushed, and he seemed anxious and fearful. The staff recognized Mr. Morgan from a previous admission some months before. At that time, he had been admitted during the early stages of delirium tremens (alcohol withdrawal delirium). He had experienced grossly elevated blood pressure and frightening hallucinations about being attacked by rats. However, after completion of detoxification, Mr. Morgan signed himself out and did not enter the rehabilitation treatment program offered at the center. He denied drinking other than socially, commenting, "I just have a few beers at the end of the day to relax." Mr. Morgan was immediately admitted. Meanwhile Mrs. Morgan offered further information. "He almost hit that kid this morning. Thank goodness it was the bicycle and not the kid that was crumpled! I've had it—no more covering up, no more calling work to say he is 'sick.' I think he really tried to quit drinking the last time he left the center but couldn't. Now he's probably going to lose his job. David's a math teacher and the principal called last week to tell me that he's given David his last warning about drinking. David never told me, but kids have been complaining that he's drinking during school, and parents have been calling in. I've always let David blame me for his drinking, for nagging him. I finally told my sister, and she says maybe I am part of the fault, but for a different reason—because I continue to accept David's excuses and help him cover up. Now, this morning, he almost hit that kid. I'm so scared! I love him, and I'll stick around *this* time. But if he signs himself out, I'm through!"

THE ESSENTIAL COMPONENTS OF A PLAN OF CARE FOR A CLIENT WITH BEHAVIOR RELATED TO ALCOHOL ABUSE

STRENGTHS: Intelligent, supportive wife

Revision Date: Insert date

DATE	NEED/PROBLEM	GOALS — ACTIVE GOALS	MAINTENANCE GOALS	APPROACH
Insert date	**1.** Temporary problem (T.P.): Intoxication related to excessive ingestion of alcohol, as evidenced by slurred speech, flushed face, unsteady gait, smell of alcohol, anxiety, fearfulness	**1a.** Mr. Morgan will improve physically and be able to care for self, in 1 to 3 days (Insert date)		Admit to detoxification room (well-lighted, uncluttered, easy observation, quiet) for 1 to 3 days. Position on side to prevent aspiration from possible vomiting. Reposition every 2 hours, more often if needed. Visually check client every 15 minutes. Based on previous admission history, monitor carefully for signs of impending D.T.'s. Monitor and record vital signs every 2 hours for first 12 hours, then 4 times a day for the next 3 days (unless elevated) and every day for the next 4 days. Administer medication as ordered for one or more of the objective symptoms: —Elevated B.P. (i.e., above 140/90) —Elevated pulse (i.e., above 90) —Diaphoresis —Hallucinations —Seizures or history of seizures during withdrawal —Agitation Check vital signs 2 hours after each dose of medication is given. Contact physician for further direction if vital signs do not stabilize after usual dose of medication. Reorient client as needed. Offer one cup juice every hour (likes grape and cranberry juice).
Insert date		**1b.** Mr. Morgan will verbalize that he is		Assist with feeding, as needed initially.

Table continues on following page.

THE ESSENTIAL COMPONENTS OF A PLAN OF CARE FOR A CLIENT WITH BEHAVIOR RELATED TO ALCOHOL ABUSE—*Continued*

STRENGTHS: Intelligent, supportive wife

Revision Date: Insert date

DATE	NEED/PROBLEM	GOALS		APPROACH
		ACTIVE GOALS	**MAINTENANCE GOALS**	
		less anxious and fearful, within 8 to 12 hours (Insert date and time)		Assist with personal hygiene, as needed. (Meet physical needs.) Be aware of personal attitudes. Mr. Morgan tends to exaggerate signs of rejection. Responds to one-to-one contacts and reassurance.
Insert date	2. Impaired functioning in job performance and personal relationships related to drinking, as indicated by almost hitting the paper boy with car, threat of losing job, threat of wife leaving him if he does not complete treatment successfully	2. Mr. Morgan will actively involve himself in planning and following through on a structured plan for change to quit drinking, beginning in 5 days (Insert date)		Review the program with Mr. Morgan; request input; personalize the program, and explain that deviation from the program is not permitted. Give Mr. Morgan a copy of the program. The program will include: —Personal goal planning —Group meeting to deal with denial, dependency, values clarification, self-esteem, relaxation techniques —Lectures and films on alcoholism per daily schedule —A.A. lessons per daily schedule —Participation in occupational therapy and recreational goal-directed activities —Participation in recreation therapy for leisure counseling and participation in recreational activities within Mr. Morgan's financial means are possibilities for follow-through. (Likes bowling.) —Contact vocational services counselor for an in-house job to provide spending money, responsibility, and satisfaction. —Attend nutrition class specific to relationship of nutrition and alcohol.

THE ESSENTIAL COMPONENTS OF A PLAN OF CARE FOR A CLIENT WITH BEHAVIOR RELATED TO ALCOHOL ABUSE—*Continued*

STRENGTHS: Intelligent, supportive wife

Revision Date: Insert date

DATE	NEED/PROBLEM	GOALS		APPROACH
		ACTIVE GOALS	MAINTENANCE GOALS	
				—Attend counseling sessions one time per week with Mrs. Morgan. (Provide structure, information and personal growth.)
Insert date	3. Attempts at manipulating staff, as evidenced by request for extra medication	3. Mr. Morgan will stop asking for extra medication not indicated for his physical condition, within 5 days (Insert date)		Evaluate request for medications by taking vital signs. When medication is not needed, offer natural ways to relieve tension, such as warm shower or bath, physical activity. (Offer positive ways to cope.)
Insert date	4. Inability to maintain sobriety, as evidenced by continuation of drinking after last discharge		4. After discharge, Mr. Morgan will maintain sobriety in his home and work setting on a continuing basis with support.	Attend weekly, community, open A.A. meeting twice with other clients and staff. Attend closed A.A. meetings after discharge, starting day of discharge. Continue weekly counseling sessions for six weeks after discharge with Mrs. Morgan. Encourage Mrs. Morgan to seek help through Al-Anon. Encourage continuation of hobbies and recreational activities involved in while an inpatient. Encourage practicing relaxation techniques daily to lower anxiety level naturally. (Advance planning to maintain sobriety after discharge through education and support.)

References for Unit III

About Suicide, 1979 Greenfield, ME, Channing L. Bete Co., Inc.

Alcoholics Anonymous, 1952. Twelve Steps and Twelve Traditions. New York, AA Publishing, Inc.

American Psychological Association, 1980. Diagnostic and Statistical Manual of Mental Disorders. 3rd ed. Washington, D.C., The American Psychological Association.

Bartel, M., 1979. Non-verbal communication in patients with Alzheimer's disease. J Gerontol Nurs, Vol. 5, No. 4, July-August, pp. 21–31.

Blum, E.M., and Blum, R.H., 1967. Alcoholism. San Francisco, Jossey-Bass Inc., Publishers.

Burgess, A., 1981. Psychiatric Nursing in the Hospital and the Community. 3rd ed. Englewood Cliffs, NJ, Prentice-Hall, Inc.

Burkhalter, P.K., 1975. Nursing Care of the Alcoholic and Drug Abuser. New York, McGraw-Hill Book Company.

Caton, C., 1981. The new chronic patient and the system of community care. Hosp Community Psychiatry, Vol. 32, No. 7, July, pp. 475–478.

Drye, R., Goulding, R.L., and Goulding, M., 1973. No-suicide decisions: Patient monitoring of suicidal risk. Am J Psychiatry, Vol. 130, No. 2, February, pp. 171–174.

Estes, N.J., Smith-DiJulio, K., and Heinemann, M.E., 1980. Nursing Diagnosis of the Alcoholic Person. St. Louis, The C.V. Mosby Co.

Expert Committee on Mental Health, 1951. First report of the alcoholism subcommittee. WHO Technical Report Series No. 42. Geneva, World Health Organization.

Frederick, C.J., 1976. Trends in mental health self-destructive behavior among younger age groups. Rockville, MD, NIMH, Department of Health, Education, and Welfare.

Grossman, H.J., 1977. A Manual on Terminology and Classification in Mental Retardation. 3rd ed. Washington, D.C., American Association on Mental Deficiency.

Hendin, H., 1982. Suicide in America. New York, W.W. Norton.

Horoshak, I., 1977. How to Spot and Handle High-Risk Patients. R.N., Vol. 40, No. 9, September, pp. 58–63.

Husain, S.A., and Vandiver, T., 1984. Suicide in Children and Adolescents. New York, Spectrum Publications, Inc.

Irving, S., 1983. Basic Psychiatric Nursing. 3rd ed. Philadelphia, W.B. Saunders Co.

Jacobson, G.R., 1976. The Alcoholisms: Detection, Assessment, and Diagnosis. New York, Human Sciences Press.

Johnson, V.E., 1973. I'll Quit Tomorrow. New York, Harper and Row Publishers, Inc.

Klagsbrun, F., 1976. Too Young To Die. Boston, Houghton Mifflin Co.

Lamb, H., 1982. Young adult chronic patients: The new drifters. Hosp Community Psychiatry, Vol. 33, No. 6, June, pp. 465–468.

Lipowski, Z.J., 1980. A new look at organic brain syndrome. Am J Psychiatry, Vol. 137, No. 6, June, pp. 674–678.

Macky, A., 1983. OBS and nursing care. J Gerontol Nurs, Vol. 9, No. 2, February, pp. 74–79, 83–85.

Maslow, A., 1970. Motivation and Personality. 2nd ed. New York, Harper and Row Publishers, Inc.

Payne, D., and Clunn, P., 1977. Psychiatric Mental Health Nursing. 2nd ed. New York, Medical Examination Publishing Company, Inc.

Pepper, B., Kirshner, M., and Ryglewicz H., 1981. The young adult chronic patient: Overview of a population. Hosp Community Psychiatry, Vol. 32, No. 7, July, pp. 463–469.

Perko, J., and Kreigh, H., 1983. Psychiatric and Mental Health Nursing: A Commitment to Care and Concern. 2nd ed. Reston, Va., Reston Publishing Company, Inc.

Pothier, P., 1980. Psychiatric Nursing. Boston, Little, Brown and Co.

Pyke, J., 1982. Dependency issues in long-term treatment of schizophrenia. Issues Ment Health Nurs, Vol. 4, pp. 77–85.

Rabkin, B., 1979. Growing Up Dead. Nashville, Abingdon Publishing Co.

Reisberg, B., and Ferris, S., 1982. Diagnosis and assessment of the older patient. Hosp Community Psychiatry, Vol. 33, No. 2, February, pp. 104–110.

Richardson, K., 1982. Hope and flexibility. Nursing '82, June, pp. 65–69.

Rudden, M., Gilmore, M., and Frances, A., 1982. Delusion: When to confront the facts of life. Am J Psychiatry, Vol. 137, No. 7, July, pp. 929–931.

Schneidman, E., and Farberow, N.L. (eds.), 1957. Clues to Suicide. New York, McGraw-Hill Book Company, Inc.

Schwartz, S., and Goldfinger, S., 1981. The new chronic patient: Clinical characteristics of an emerging subgroup. Hosp Community Psychiatry, Vol. 32, No. 7, July, pp. 470–474.

Sibert, S., 1983. Ethics in psychosocial nursing. J Psychosocial Nurs, Vol. 21, No. 12, December, pp. 29–33.

Silverstein, L.M., 1977. Consider the Alternative. Minneapolis, Comp Care Publications.

Steiner, C., 1971. Games Alcoholics Play: The Analysis of Life Scripts. New York, Grove Press, Inc.

Swift, R.M., How to Help An Alcoholic Who Insists He Doesn't Need Any Help. Westport, Ct., Fairfield County Council on Alcoholism, Inc.

Valles, J., 1965. How To Live With An Alcoholic. New York, Simon & Schuster, Inc.

Wilson, H., and Kneisl, C., 1979. Psychiatric Nursing. Massachusetts, Addison-Wesley Publishing Co.

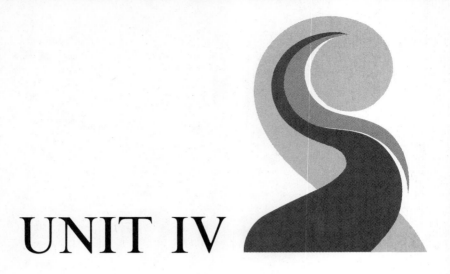

UNIT IV

HEALTH PROVIDERS AND INTERVENTIONS

INDIVIDUAL APPROACH

LEARNING OBJECTIVES—Upon completing this chapter, the reader will be able to:

1. Give two questions the health provider can use to determine personal reasons for working with an emotionally disturbed client.

2. Describe techniques of effective listening.

3. Give one example of when "I" messages are used.

4. Discuss the significance of nonverbal communication clues.

5. Explain the difference between assertiveness, nonassertiveness, and aggressiveness.

6. Monitor his interactions with the client using the evaluation exercise in Unit VI.

KNOWING YOURSELF

An essential key to the effectiveness of care depends on the health provider's self-understanding. Unless the provider knows himself, gets in touch with his feelings, and understands his reactions to those feelings and how they influence others' behavior, the provider can sabotage the best developed plans for client care.

When working with the emotionally disturbed, the health provider can become the immediate target of a barrage of negative, hostile, and aggressive emotions and of problems that are difficult for the strongest to cope with. If, however, the provider has examined and continues to examine his life, and feels reasonably secure and adequate—is at least aware of vulnerable spots—the provider will not be unduly disturbed by a client's anger, criticism, and resentment or by the client's need for warmth and closeness. The provider will realize that while these feelings are displaced onto him, they are not aroused by him but by events in the client's past. Then the provider will be free to see the client as he really is, to understand and tolerate the client's behavior, and to work constructively with the client—a therapeutic course of action that will reinforce the sense of worthiness basic to the client's recovery.

If, on the contrary, the health provider has not taken stock of himself and is insecure, he will be blinded by his own feelings of inadequacy and worthlessness. If the provider continues to be afraid, unsure, and completely unaware of why he is so, he will feel threatened by the hostile client, even though the client's hostility has nothing to do with the provider, and rejected by the withdrawn client, even though the client's isolation is not of the provider's making. Then, the provider, understanding neither the client's behavior nor his reactions to it, will respond defensively, with anger, browbeating, belittling, or distance. This pathological course of action will, in turn, reinforce the client's low self-image, which is part of the client's illness (Let Your Light So Shine, 1968:12).

The health provider must feel secure enough to respond appropriately and therapeutically to clients' behavior. The following is a list of questions the provider can ask himself in order to gain more self-awareness:

A. What are my motivations?
—Do I honestly want to help?
—Do I feel I have the capacity for it and the endurance?
—Does it have value for me?
—Can I give, or must I always be on the receiving end?
—What are my reasons for choosing this work? To compete with someone else? To get rid of hidden guilt by caring for others?

"Unconscious motivations, unrecognized, can defeat conscious goals" (Let Your Light So Shine, 1968:12).

B. Why do I feel as I do?
—If I feel inadequate, inferior, and unsure of myself, are these feelings realistic, or am I more competent than I allow myself to believe?
—Why can't I tolerate a client's display of warmth and affection?
—Why can't I show warmth in return?
—Why am I so threatened?
—Why do I feel compelled to keep my distance?
—Why do I make it difficult for the client to say "Thank you"?
C. What are my emotional needs?
—Do I require sympathy, protection, and warmth so much that I err by being too sympathetic, too protective, too warm toward the client. Or, do I fear closeness so much that I err by being indifferent, rejecting, cold?
—Do I have an excessive need to be liked, to be constantly reassured? If so, I may be angry when the client I am helping is rude, unappreciative.
—Do I cover up feelings of inferiority with a mask of superiority? If so, I may reject the client who has similar feelings, although his real need is to be accepted.
—Do I disguise feelings of inadequacy by being dictatorial, laying down the law? If so, I may prevent the client from getting close, and my rigidity may stifle the client's emotional growth.
—Do I need to feel important, liked at any cost? If so, do I unconsciously keep people dependent upon me?
D. What are my prejudices?
—Do I react to the client as an individual or with preconceived ideas passed on from my parents, my co-workers, or the label the client wears?
—Can I justify my prejudices? Or, are they derogatory feelings that get in the way of a warm relationship? (Let Your Light So Shine, 1968:13).

If such self-examination is difficult, even painful, take comfort from Harry Stack Sullivan's words: ". . . no one has grave difficulties in living if he has a very good grasp on what is happening to him" (Sullivan, 1954:24).

The following poem by a practical nursing student shows how she got to know herself, using the problem-solving approach.

ANXIETY ABOUT MENTAL ILLNESS

Anxiety, no don't do it,
don't turn that knob and go through.
Manic depression, hallucinations,
schizo, suicidal, it just might get to
you.

I don't want that trip, I don't
want that fear.
Just turn that knob, look,
oh no, it's all right here.
I don't understand, can't comprehend, don't know how to help them mend.
Seclusion room, zig zagging,
banging in the wall, slashing wrists,
alcohol and pills, will it ever end?
Anxiety, no don't turn that
knob, don't walk on through that door.

Sitting in the classroom, thoughts
run through my mind.
Words, symptoms, approach, I don't
know enough to help her.
Will I do more harm, put her
further behind?
If she throws me a suicide
clue, will I catch it? Yes,
I could do that, but will I say
what's right, to help her through it?
Helplessness, insecurity, Why
don't I feel more sure, way inside
me?
I'm trying too hard, but the
mind's so delicate.
I want to learn so much more
before I dive into it.
I'll only take it as far as I already know.

This morning, anxiety
came again.
It lasted for a little while
but it didn't win.
The one I was afraid of, was
more afraid of me.
I listened and observed, and
tomorrow I'll approach and talk.
Probably when he's going
down the hall for a walk.
I didn't know what to say
and how to approach.
Instead of helping, I felt like
an intruder.
Quietly sitting beside him,
I thought it all out.
Then I told him in my own
words what it was about.
I didn't push, I let him
lead.
He knew I was there to talk
with when he had the need.

We got to know each other
just a little bit.
He's starting to reach out, I can
feel it.
Tomorrow I'll try one to one.
Either playing cards or working on puzzles. I'll get an approach
begun.

My final chapter is really
a new beginning.
I solved my fears, I didn't
lose, but ended up winning.
I faced it, erased it, and
I grew.
I achieved so much more
than I thought I would.
I was so scared and frightened,
I never thought I could.
I feel proud, not so much
for myself, but that I actually
touched some people along my
struggling road.
That's what really makes
me feel great, I really did
some good while I was
growing myself.
I'll use what I learned and
go on to grow.
I started with a box full of
pieces.
I dumped them out, spread
them all around.
Started with the border, as good
a start as any.
But now to fit in the
middle, the pieces are so many.
Nurse-client relationships,
caring, accepting, listening.
I'm almost done.
Now I see what it's about;
A student who was afraid,
and insecure, who grew by
facing, erasing and starting
brand new.
Pieces in the box, put
together as a whole.
Made me someone I'm
proud to know.

BONNIE KAMINSKI, L.P.N.

COMMUNICATION SKILLS

The following statements suggest that communication is a complex process involving many skills:

"I know you believe you understand what you think I said. But I am not sure you realize that what you heard is not what I meant."
"If you really want to understand me, please hear what I am not saying, what I may never be able to say."
"You can't expect to talk straight if you think in circles."
"If there's anything I can't stand, it's someone who talks while I'm interrupting."
"If you do not understand my silence, you will not understand my words."
"Listen hard. You may hear something you never heard before."
"Speak kind words and you will hear kind echoes."
"Don't just talk. Say something."

Communication involves the exchange of attitudes, feelings, and ideas; and a full understanding of the other person's position. Therefore, many messages are shared both verbally and nonverbally. These messages include:
—What you *actually* say.
—What you *think* you said.
—What the other person actually *hears.*
—What the other person *thinks* he hears.
—What the other person *says.*
—What you *think* the other person said.

Source Unknown

Active Listening

Growth is fostered through communication. This is done by allowing persons to own their problems. The focus of this section will be on the skills involved in this process. The skill most used in allowing a person to own his problem is *active listening.* Active listening is a method of influencing an individual to find his own solution to his problems (Gordon, 1970:66). The health provider who receives the message from the client, who is the sender, must demonstrate verbal and nonverbal behaviors that convey acceptance, understanding, and confidence that the client can think through his problem and come to conclusions and answers on his own (Norton, 1978:118). In receiving the message, the health provider tries to understand what the client is feeling or what the client's message means. The provider then puts this understanding into his own words and reflects it back for the client's verification/clarification. The provider needs to determine with the client whether the return message or feedback was accurate and clear. The goal of the provider in active listening is to always keep the door open.

The client is thwarted in his effort to own and solve his problem if the provider sends a message of his own, such as:
—An order or command
  "You must eat."
—A threat
  "If you don't take your bath, you can't go to the birthday party."
—A moral obligation
  "It is your duty to take care of yourself."
—A lecture or argument
  "The facts are . . ."

"Here is why you are wrong . . ."
—A criticism or judgment
"You are not thinking straight."
"You are lazy."
—An evaluation or compliment
"You've done a good job."
"That's a very good drawing."
—Advice or suggestion
"If I were you, I would . . ."
"Why don't you . . ."
—An interpretation
"You're just trying to get attention by . . ."
—Reassurance
"Everything will be all right."
—A probing question
"Now why would you think that I don't like you?"

"Questions are incomplete, indirect, veiled, impersonal, and, consequently, ineffective messages that often breed defensive reactions and resistance" (Lalanne, 1975:134).

Consider the classic parent/child exchange:

Where did you go? — Out
What did you do? — Nothing

The exchange illustrates how ineffective questions may be. The most ineffective question is one that begins with "Why," since it is usually followed by "because." The "why–because" interaction leads to an endless chain of futile questions and fruitless answers that take one further away from a solution to the problem.

All of these messages close the door to active listening because they attempt to solve the problem for the client. In doing so, the provider conveys to the client that he has found the client's behavior unacceptable, and, therefore, the provider is solving the problem for the client.

EXAMPLE

Client to Health Provider:	"I don't know whether to go out and look for a job first or get a place to live."
Health Provider (closing door):	"If I were you, I would certainly get a job before looking for a place to live."
Health Provider (keeping the door open):	"It sounds as though you are having difficulty in deciding which is more important to do first, look for a job or a place to live!"

Active listening can be risky. To be open to the feelings, ideas, and attitudes of another can be threatening, unless the health provider is willing to be flexible, to change, and to be human (Gordon, 1970:61). This is why "knowing thyself" is so important. The alternative is defensive behavior that blocks effective communication. "As a person becomes more and more defensive, he becomes less and less able to perceive accurately the motives, the values, and the emotions of the sender" (Gibb, 1982:14). The following poem conveys clearly what active listening truly is:

LISTEN

When I ask you to listen to me
  and you start giving advice,
  you have not done what I asked.

When I ask you to listen to me
  and you begin to tell me why I shouldn't feel that way,
  you are trampling on my feelings.

When I ask you to listen to me
  and you feel you have to do something to solve my problem,
  you have failed me, strange as that may seem.

Listen! All I asked, was that you listen.
  not talk or do—just hear me.
Advice is cheap: 25 cents will get you both Dear Abby and
  Billy Graham in the same newspaper.
And I can do for myself; I'm not helpless;
  Maybe discouraged and faltering, but not helpless.

When you do something for me that I can and need to do
  for myself, you contribute to my fear and weakness.

But, when you accept as a simple fact that I do feel what I feel,
  no matter how irrational, then I can quit trying to convince
  you and can get about the business of understanding what's
  behind this irrational feeling.
  And when that's clear, the answers are obvious and I
  don't need advice.
Irrational feelings make sense when we understand what's
  behind them.

Perhaps that's why prayer works, sometimes, for some people
  because God is mute, and he doesn't give advice or
  try to fix things. "They" just listen and let you
  work it out for yourself.

So, please listen and just hear me. And, if you want to
  talk, wait a minute for your turn; and I'll listen to you.

ANONYMOUS

"I" MESSAGES

When a client's behavior is a problem to the health provider because it is interfering in some tangible way with the satisfying of a provider's need, then the provider owns the problem (Gordon, 1970:64). When owning the problem, the provider uses "I" messages in communicating. "I" messages are clear and honest statements of fact about the provider. On the other hand, "You" messages are client-oriented and, therefore, make the client feel defensive. "You know" means everyone knows. "You" statements can be made fairly easily because such statements do not involve the revelation of self.

The underlying theme in communication is to allow individuals to own their problems. If the client is to own his problem, then the health provider uses active listening.

If the provider owns the problem, then "I" messages are used. If a client is too confused or has organic brain impairment that limits his problem-solving abilities, then the provider must communicate in simple, clear "I" statements. For example, "I want you to eat now," or "I am going to give you a bath now," rather than, "You should eat," or "Do you want to take a bath?" The latter two interactions usually bring negative results.

As previously mentioned, communication is verbal and nonverbal. Verbal communication includes the oral and written word; however, nonverbal communication is more extensive, including more than 60 percent of the information that people pass on to others (Forsyth, 1983:34). Components of nonverbal communication include appearance, movement, eye contact, posture, facial expression, gestures, and touch—personal space, what is frequently referred to as body language. Sometimes the nonverbal message contradicts the verbal message and is the source of the well-known cliche, "Actions speak louder than words." Karl Jaspers, in *The Perennial Scope of Philosophy*, emphasizes the importance of communication as follows (Jaspers, 1949:182):

> Communication in every form is so much a part of man as man in the very depth of his being, that it must always remain possible and one can never know how far it will go.

Assertiveness versus Aggressiveness

Assertiveness, not aggressiveness, is a required characteristic of the vitally committed client advocate. Assertiveness, according to Webster's dictionary, is characterized by taking a positive stand, being confident in your statement, or being positive in a persistent way. The health provider works in a setting that requires speaking frankly and openly to others in such a way that the rights of others are not violated. While it is not the provider's right to hurt others deliberately, it is unrealistic to be inhibited to the point of never hurting anyone. Some people are hurt because they are unreasonably sensitive, and some use their sensitivity to manipulate others. The provider has the right to express thoughts and feelings. To do otherwise would be insincere and would deny the clients and other staff the opportunity to learn to deal with their feelings. Assertiveness, then, is a way of expressing oneself without insulting another person. It communicates respect for the other person, although not necessarily for the other person's behavior.

Three rules of thumb are helpful in being assertive:

1. Own your feelings; that is, do not blame others for the way you feel. For example:
   Positive—"I feel angry because you continue to be late for work without notifying the unit."
   Negative—"You make me mad because you're always late."
2. Make your feelings known by being direct and by beginning your statements with "I". For example:
   Positive—"I find your referring to the client by diagnosis very annoying."
   Negative—"You shouldn't call the client by his diagnosis."
3. Be sure that your nonverbal communication matches your verbal message. For example:
   Positive—"I want you to take your hand off my leg" (said in a serious tone of voice and with a serious expression).
   Negative—"You shouldn't put your hand there" (accompanied by a smile).

Outspoken people are often automatically considered assertive when, in reality, their lack of consideration for others may characterize aggressive behavior. Aggressive behavior violates the rights of others. It is an attack on the person rather than on the person's behavior. "Early in life, the person with aggressive behavior acquires a peculiar sensitivity to situations in which he experiences inadequacy, a strong sense of rejection, and in which he expects punishment" (Irving, 1978:69). The purpose of aggressive behavior is to dominate or put the other person down. The behavior, while expressive, is self-defeating, as it quickly distances the health provider from other staff and clients.

Another self-defeating behavior is nonassertive (passive) behavior. Nonassertive behavior is dishonest. The nonassertive person does not express his own feelings and needs when his rights are infringed upon deliberately or accidently. "His attitude toward himself is self-depreciatory, and he experiences marked insecurity in his relationships with other people" (Irving, 1978:70). By not taking the risk and not being honest, he typically feels hurt, misunderstood, and often angry. Since he does not allow his needs to be known, he is the loser. The assertive client is rare. More commonly, we see the aggressive, demanding client or the nonassertive client who has difficulty asking directly about his illness, medications, and therapies. Clients feel even more powerless in an institutional setting and do not see themselves as equal to the health provider. Childish, noncompliant behaviors may emerge and need to be recognized as the client's attempt to maintain some control. "Noncompliance may be a natural effort by patients to regain mastery over the situation" (Jenkins, 1982:59). Many clients can benefit from having the health provider teach them how to be appropriately assertive. Jenkins (1982:51–63) suggests that suicidal, alcoholic, depressed, and withdrawn clients are potential candidates for assertiveness training.

According to Jenkins (1982:59), a suicidal tendency in some mentally ill clients may represent "the only way for these individuals to release pent-up aggression and to assert control over the nature of the expression." Once the initial crisis has been dealt with, the health provider has a good opportunity to listen to the client and to begin to work with him on healthy ways of asserting himself.

Another form of self-destructive behavior related to nonassertive behavior is alcoholism. Brown and Ostrow (1980:328) discovered that "Non-assertive behavior sets up our patients for a drinking episode . . . patients will note that it is only when drunk that they are able to express anger and emotions built up as a result of passive behavior. Drinking, then, may be the end result of a series of unexpressed emotions." Once again the health provider has an excellent opportunity to work with the alcoholic client to help him learn to express assertively his emotions to those of significance in his life.

Assertive techniques are also useful for the client suffering from depressive or withdrawal patterns of behavior. The depressed client tends to accept his view of hopelessness and helplessness as being real. The client with a withdrawal pattern of behavior finds it difficult, initially, to accept a relationship with the health provider. It takes great skill and persistence on the part of the provider to develop a trusting relationship with either of these clients. Once the relationship is established, the provider can teach the client assertive techniques that will enhance his self-esteem. The provider's own attitudes and use of aggressive, assertive, and nonassertive responses are of major importance in dealing with the client. Some providers are rejecting toward clients who know and assert their needs. The provider must evaluate personal responses to the client and be aware that aggressive or nonassertive responses may negate the effect of well-planned treatment goals. The client may also emulate the negative behavior modeled for him. Assertive behavior that is honest behavior is essential in meeting the client's needs.

CLIENT'S RIGHTS AND RESPONSIBILITIES

In 1972, the American Hospital Association presented a Patient's Bill of Rights. The Bill included 12 provisions that would ensure more effective client care. The areas addressed in the Bill of Rights included the client's right to respectful care, complete information about his condition, informed consent, refusal of treatment, privacy, confidentiality, hospital services that he requests, information about the hospital's affiliation with other institutions, refusal of experimental treatment, continuity of care, information about his bill, and knowledge of the hospital's rules and regulations that apply to his conduct (Patient's Bill of Rights, 1973:29). States began to use these rights as a basis for developing laws that would protect the client's legal rights. In Kansas, modifications were made so that the rights would protect clients admitted to a psychiatric hospital (Patient's Bill of Rights:32–34).

With every right there is a responsibility. Some of a client's responsibilities that are related to his or her rights include asking questions, respecting others, planning carefully, giving full information, following physician's/hospital's instructions, reporting any changes, keeping appointments, and paying bills promptly, if at all possible (What You Should Know About Patients' Rights, 1982:10–11).

The following examples of a health provider's interactions with a client emphasize the application of some of the provisions of the Patient's Bill of Rights. The right being applied appears in parentheses.

Health Provider's Interactions That Enhance The Human Dignity Of The Client

HEALTH PROVIDER'S INTERACTIONS	CLIENT'S REACTION
1. Recognizing the client's presence (respectful care) *Example:* Health provider is talking at the desk when Tom approaches. Provider acknowledges Tom by saying, "Is there something that I can help you with, Tom?"	Client feels that he counts.
2. Listening to what the client has to say (respectful care) *Example:* "You were telling me, Joe, about what you did on the week-end. I would like to hear more about your activities."	Client feels that what he has to say is important.
3. Allowing the client to *own* his problem (respectful care) *Example:* Client—"What should I do first, take a bath or clean my room?" Provider—"It sounds as though you are having difficulty in setting priorities."	Client feels that he has some control over his life; he can make decisions.
4. Referring to clients by their proper name and title (respectful care) *Example:* "Mr. Jones (instead of Grandpa), are you going out today?"	Client feels that he has a separate identity.
5. Being consistent in the care that is given the client (continuity of care) *Example:* Follow the care plan that has been developed for the client. If you don't agree with the plan of care, do not change it on your own; instead, request a care plan meeting.	Client develops a sense of security and direction. He knows that he can depend on certain consequences if he performs certain behaviors.
6. Relating to clients as adults (unless working with children) (respectful care) *Example:* "I want you to take a bath before supper." (Instead of "You should . . .")	Client receives clear directions and does not feel put-down.
7. Limits are set for the client's benefit and not the provider's convenience (respectful care) *Example:* "I want you to go to your room. I'll be there in 5 minutes to see if you've gained control of your behavior."	Client receives positive, fair directions without a threat, eliminating the need to test the limit.
8. Focusing on the strengths of the client. Giving credit for positive behavior. Simple decisions may be major decisions for the client and represent a strength. (respectful care) *Example:* "I'm pleased to see that you made the decision to wash your hair today."	Client feels useful and significant and gets the message that he can make decisions about his life.

Health Provider's Interactions That Enhance The Human Dignity Of The Client—
Continued

HEALTH PROVIDER'S INTERACTIONS	CLIENT'S REACTION
9. Allowing client to do as much as possible for himself, depending on the fluctuations in his condition. The client will live up to the expectations of others. (respectful care) *Example:* "You seem stronger today, Mr. Jones. I want you to feed yourself."	Client feels that he is improving and can be more independent.
10. Trusting the client's desire to find more positive behaviors than he has at this time (respectful care) *Example:* "I know that you want to control your behavior, but right now you need some help from me."	Client feels that the provider trusts him. Provider's positive attitude communicates a sense of hope.
11. Promising only what you can carry out. Determine in advance if unsure that you can carry through on promise. (complete information) *Example:* "I've checked on my schedule, and I'll be here tomorrow, so I will take you to the store then."	Client feels that he can depend on the provider.
12. Holding the client responsible for his behavior (knowledge of hospital regulations) *Example:* "When you made the decision to run away, you knew what the consequences of your actions would be."	Client develops a sense of responsibility and learns to view limits set as consequences of his behavior rather than punishment.

A violation of client's rights can be dehumanizing and abusive. The following are examples of such behaviors:

Health Provider's Interactions That Are Dehumanizing To The Client

HEALTH PROVIDER'S INTERACTIONS	CLIENT'S REACTION
1. Talking about the client in his presence. *Example:* Saying to the family member who is returning client from a week-end pass, "Did Joey behave himself while he was home?"	Makes client feel like an object.
2. Reminding a client that he will not do something negative, such as hit another person. *Example:* "You'd better not hit anyone today!"	Client is being set up to act out. This is reinforcement of the negative behavior.
3. Threatening client (showing who is "boss"). *Example:* "If you give me any trouble today, I'll put you in the Geri-chair."	Client complies through fear.
4. Conversing with another health provider instead of the client while caring for the client. *Example:* While health providers are giving their respective clients a bath, one says to the other, "I really had a blast this week-end."	Client feels that he doesn't exist, is a nobody.
5. Referring to a client by room number or diagnosis. *Example:* "I have that new 'schizophrenic' today."	Client feels like a nonperson.
6. Disregarding the client's plan of care and doing your "own thing." *Example:* "I don't know who came up with	Client is confused as to what is expected of him and becomes more insecure because the rules keep changing.

Table continues on following page.

Health Provider's Interactions That Are Dehumanizing To The Client—*Continued*

HEALTH PROVIDER'S INTERACTIONS	CLIENT'S REACTION
that dumb rule. Of course you can go home this week-end."	
7. Repeating what the client says in a mimicky way. *Example:* "I want to go home. I want to go home . . ." (over and over).	Client feels that he doesn't have anything of worth to say; is afraid to express himself.
8. Not listening to clients. *Example:* "Oh, don't worry about that; we'll take care of you."	Client feels that no one understands him or cares.
9. Lining clients up and then making them wait for the activity. *Example:* Calling clients together to leave the unit for a walk and then saying, "I'm not ready to go yet."	This can provoke anger in the client.
10. Demeaning, discounting, or belittling clients. *Example:* "What's the point of walking her? She's never going to leave here."	The client feels hopeless and helpless—a sense of being trapped.
11. Teasing clients. *Example:* "Maybe I won't give you your cigarettes this time."	The client feels put down.
12. Treating clients as children. *Example:* Not giving a client available chores. Doing all of a client's care, though he is capable of doing some of it himself. Diapering clients who could be bowel and bladder trained. Talking to clients in baby talk. Using "should" and "can't" in speaking to clients.	Clients feel as though they no longer have control over their own lives. They have lost their "power base."
13. Provoking guilt in clients. *Example:* "How can you be like that? Your daughter does so much for you."	This can cause the client to become depressed or outwardly angry.
14. Ridiculing clients. *Example:* "Can't you ever do things right?" or "Look how dirty you are. Can't you keep yourself clean?"	Client feels he has failed and can't possibly succeed.
15. Exploiting clients. *Example:* Using the client who is mentally retarded as a watchdog. "Let me know when the supervisor is coming."	Clients feel used.
16. Flirting with clients. *Example:* "Gee, honey, when are we going out?" If client reaches out in a sexual way, he is referred to as a "dirty old man."	Client perceives behavior as genuine and is confused by health provider's response.
17. Displacing your angry feelings onto clients. *Example:* Yelling at clients; shouting directions; rough handling of clients.	Client becomes fearful of expressing his needs because of the danger of retaliation.
18. Clowning around in the presence of clients who are confused and disoriented. While a sense of humor is valuable, it is important that the expression of humor be relevant to the situation. *Example:* Health providers joke with each other about occurrences in their personal lives that are not related to the work setting.	Client becomes more confused by the environmental stimulation, which can trigger aggressive outbursts.
19. Showing favoritism to selected clients. *Example:* "I brought my favorite girl a piece of candy today."	Other clients become jealous, begin to act out.

REFERENCES

Alberti, R.E., and Emmons, M.L., 1974. Your Perfect Right: A Guide To Assertive Behavior. 2nd ed. San Luis Obispo, CA, Impact Publishers, Inc.

Berger, M.M., 1977. Working With People Called Patients. New York, Brunner/Mazel, Publishers.

Bloom, L.Z., Coburn, K., and Pearlman, J., 1975. The New Assertive Woman. New York, Delacorte Press.

Brown, L.S., and Ostrow, F., 1980. The development of an assertiveness program on an alcoholic unit. Int J Addict, Vol. 15, p. 324.

Clark, H.H., 1974. The power of positive speaking. Psychol Today, November, pp. 102, 108–111.

Davis, K., 1972. Human Behavior at Work: Human Relations and Organizational Behavior. New York, McGraw-Hill Book Company.

Forsyth, D., 1983. Looking good to communicate better with patients. Nursing '83, July, pp. 34–37.

Gibb, J.R., 1982. Defensive communication. J Nurs Adm, April, pp. 14–17.

Gordon, T., 1970. P.E.T. Parent Effectiveness Training. New York, Peter H. Wyden, Inc.

Jenkins, L.M., 1984. The concepts of assertion: From theory to practice. Issues Ment Health Nurs, Vol. 4, No. 1, January–February, pp. 51–63.

Karshmer, J.F., 1982. Rules of thumb: Hints for the psychiatric nursing student. J Psychosoc Nurs Ment Health Serv, Vol. 20, No. 3, March, pp. 25–28.

Kreigh, H.Z., and Perko, J.E., 1979. Psychiatric and Mental Health Nursing: Commitment to Care and Concern. Reston, VA, Reston Publishing Company, Inc.

Lalanne, J., 1975. Attack by question. Psychol Today. November, p. 134.

Let Your Light So Shine. 1968 Nutley, NJ, Roche Laboratories.

Norton, C.B., 1978. Can you hear between the lines? R.N., September, pp. 117–122.

The patient's bill of rights is a 12-point lesson plan. 1973 Inserv Train Educ, October, 1973, pp. 28–35.

Peplau, H.E., 1960. Talking with patients. Am J Nurs, Vol. 60, No. 7, pp. 964–966.

Smith, M., 1975. When I Say No, I Feel Guilty. New York, The Dial Press.

Southwell, M., 1977. Listening: A successful therapeutic approach. Free Assoc, August–September, pp. 1–3.

Sullivan, H.S., 1954. The Psychiatric Interview. New York, Norton and Company.

What You Should Know About Patients' Rights. 1982. South Deerfield, MA, Channing L. Bete Co., Inc.

GROUP APPROACH

LEARNING OBJECTIVES—Upon completing this chapter, the reader will be able to:

1. Define what is meant by *group*.

2. Explain what is meant by "here and now" issues.

3. List five reasons for group work.

4. Explain each of the three phases of group work.

5. Give at least ten guidelines for conducting group sessions.

6. Describe one benefit of an admission group.

7. List two goals of a socialization group.

8. State three criteria for selecting participants in a problem-solving group.

9. Explain how reality orientation classes and 24-hour per day health provider follow-through is used in reorientating a confused client.

10. Develop one topic for a remotivation session using the five basic steps.

11. Discuss two purposes of the reminiscent group.

12. Develop a sensory stimulation prop for use with a specific client.

13. Define the basic philosophy of an education group.

14. Discuss three key ideas that form the basis for client government.

DESCRIPTION OF GROUP WORK

Groups are a part of living, the primary group being the family. Within the family, attitudes and behaviors develop toward persons who have something in common, and these attitudes and behaviors influence each family member's future success in groups. According to Howe et al. (1984:1391), "A group is a congregation of three or more people who can communicate with one another to accomplish common goals. An essential feature is that the members have something in common, and this holds them together. Interaction occurs between members, and each member is influenced by the behavior and characteristics of the others and by the mood or climate present in the group."

Since World War II, group work has been a popular form of treatment with mentally ill clients. Psychiatric medication, which was introduced in the 1950s, made clients more amenable to this form of treatment. With some of the overt symptomatology under control, clients were able to share experiences and provide support to group members.

The group work described in this chapter will focus on structured groups that center on "here and now" issues. These issues offer a concrete basis for dealing with specific items the client can grasp. Such groups are led by a wide spectrum of health providers and are effective with confused and disoriented clients. Groups that focus on feelings and the dynamics behind them are categorized as psychotherapy groups. These groups are led by professionals with special training in group dynamics. The members of such groups should be able to give of themselves. On Maslow's Hierarchy of Needs (Chapter 2), they would appear at the third level, which is Love and Belongingness.

REASONS FOR GROUP WORK

Some of the reasons for group work include:

1.   The opportunity to practice alternative ways of dealing with negative feelings in a nonjudgmental, protective environment.
2.   The opportunity for a sense of belonging and acceptance.
3.   The opportunity to give as well as receive, increasing self-confidence.
4.   The opportunity for self-disclosure and the realization that others have similar feelings and problems.
5.   The opportunity to interact with others, developing greater interpersonal effectiveness.
6.   The opportunity to gain some understanding of one's feelings.
7.   The opportunity for positive reinforcement and hope for improvement.
8.   An opportunity to develop a feeling of community with others, thus decreasing the feeling of loneliness.
9.   An opportunity to realize how one's behavior affects others through peer feedback.
10.   An opportunity to transfer what is learned in the group to other situations, such as home and work.

PHASES OF GROUP WORK

To become a true group, all groups pass through set phases. The initial phase is the *introductory phase*. During this phase, group goals are clarified, and decisions are made on how to attain the goals. The communication is social, as members get to know each other. The next phase is the *active phase*. During this phase, the real work of the group takes place. The group has developed sufficient trust in each other to risk being honest and to confront each other negatively, as necessary. Clients work on attaining group goals until the time for the group to terminate has been reached. The last phase is the *closing phase*. This is a time of mixed emotions. Clients experience satisfaction in goals they have attained. They also experience the loss of support from the group that has filled a need for them during this period. It is important to have planned for this in advance by involving the client in another group, volunteer efforts, or other meaningful activity to fill the void created by the group's termination.

GUIDELINES FOR CONDUCTING GROUP SESSIONS

1.   Selection of clients should be based on certain criteria, such as similar problem, similar ability in verbal expression, emotional level, similar or varied interests.
2.   Group size is based on group goals; if clients are confused and disoriented, six to eight clients is the maximum.
3.   Select comfortable surroundings; a permanent meeting place free from distraction is desirable.

4. Acquaint oneself with clients before the group begins.

5. Briefly describe the group's purpose/goals at the beginning of the first session, such as, "We are having these meetings so that we can get to know each other better."

6. Have clients introduce themselves to each other.

7. Establish a nonthreatening and trusting climate with a statement such as, "If you don't want to contribute, that's all right."

8. Allow group members to perform tasks, such as arranging chairs, gathering materials, whatever they can do. A small, close circle promotes intimacy and cohesiveness.

9. Relate to group members with warmth and supportiveness.

10. Use verbal praise, nodding and smiling to reinforce contributions from group members.

11. Encourage group members to reinforce one another's strengths.

12. Make reluctant clients feel their ideas are wanted and needed by incorporating their contributions into the discussion.

13. Prevent talkative clients from dominating the group without feeling rejected.

14. Be patient and wait for group members to break the silence.

15. Encourage group members to direct questions to each other rather than to the leader.

16. Give power to the group by allowing them to make decisions after areas of choice have been clarified.

17. Provide for the safety of group members; guide the group away from any lengthy attack on one member.

18. Keep discussion and activity moving.

19. Listen for themes in the group, and reinforce them so that all members can be involved.

20. From time to time summarize what has been said, and ask for clarification.

21. Stimulate the group by varying techniques and format, such as role playing, films, guest leaders. Group members should participate in selecting activities.

22. The leader's attitude is contagious. If the leader is prepared and enthusiastic about group work, participants will share this enthusiasm. As a result, the composition of the group is more likely to remain stable, which in turn increases group identity and cohesiveness (Backer et al., 1978:250–264).

TYPES OF GROUP WORK

ADMISSION GROUP

The initial experience of being in a new setting can cause the client to respond in a variety of ways. A major response is that of fear—fear of what will happen to him now that the admission process is over. It would not be unusual to find out that a client facing a new admission has received his impressions about mental health facilities from movies, books, or television. A client facing a re-admission may be negatively influenced by a previous unpleasant experience. Some clients experience a sense of relief once they are away from the direct source of their problem or are reminded by a former successful experience that the mental health facility is the place to get help. It is this myriad of reactions that makes an admission group necessary during the first few post-admission days.

The admission group, sometimes known as an orientation group or newcomers group, is an open-ended group for new clients. It can be held during the day or evening, depending on scheduling. Clients usually attend this group for approximately the first week following admission, at which point they are assigned to other therapeutic programs. The group's goals are to give the new client an opportunity to express his feelings about being admitted, to ask questions about the facility, to clarify certain limits that are part of the admission, and to establish a positive relationship between clients and staff. The criterion for group selection is being newly admitted. The usual techniques used in conducting the group are open discussion and role playing. Some of the behavior clients demonstrate may appear to be a lack of cooperation or acting out. However, the behavior is related to fear and can be avoided by involving newly admitted clients in an admission group.

SOCIALIZATION GROUP

The socialization group focuses on concrete and realistic aspects of the individual and his environment. The group's goals are to stimulate the participants to begin thinking about things outside themselves and to provide them with an opportunity to talk about these things freely, promoting personal interaction between leader and client and among clients themselves. Clients chosen for this group are those whose contact with reality is tenuous, who have difficulty using their intellectual faculties, and who have difficulty interacting or socializing with others.

The group leader is, of necessity, more directive with the members of this group. This includes setting the stage for the group theme and drawing group members into the discussion. The group leader needs to prepare in advance. Suggested techniques follow:

1. Topic ideas will be most successful if they bear some relation to group members' actual interests. The group leader can get some clues for topics by talking to clients prior to the session, talking to other health providers who care for the clients, checking clients' charts in regard to previous interests and occupations, and, sometimes, talking with family members. Holidays, sports, hobbies, work, weather conditions, and pets are possible topics for beginning discussion.
2. Props, such as colorful pictures, maps, plants, tools, or a pet, when permitted, can stimulate conversation. Props, like topics, are limited only by the leader's imagination. Clients can be assigned to bring one prop of importance to them to a meeting.
3. Questions and statements by the leader may be helpful in stimulating conversation. These could include questions such as:

   a. What is the funniest thing that ever happened to you?
   b. If you could be an animal, what kind would it be and why?
   c. The holiday I remember most is _____ because _____.
   d. The first thing I remember while growing up was _____.
   e. The quality I value most about me is _____.

The physical arrangement of the room must lend itself to conversation. Arranging the chairs in a circle encourages the clients to have some physical contact with each other and places them in a position to observe others. Having juice or decaffeinated coffee available at the beginning of the session helps break the ice.

PROBLEM-SOLVING GROUP

The problem-solving process can be part of all groups, but it can also be the main focus of a group. If this is the case, the problem-solving group is open-ended and is concerned primarily with the teaching, demonstration, and implementation of the problem-solving process.

The leader of this group needs to establish a nonthreatening and trusting environment by explaining the group's purposes, which are to help the members isolate and define a problem or felt difficulty, decide on a goal, gather information pertaining to the defined problem, explore methods of solving the problem, try out one selected method, and then evaluate whether or not the method for solving the problem was successful. The leader should emphasize that the members should own their problems and that clients should direct questions to other members of the group, since in sharing information, the individual may gain some ideas about methods to consider for solving his problems. The leader should also encourage group members to reinforce one another's strengths. The leader can serve as a model for this by giving verbal praise and nodding and smiling when someone makes a contribution to the group. It is also important for the leader to guide the group away from any lengthy confrontation with one client.

Criteria for selecting clients to participate in a problem-solving group including a willingness to participate, ability to verbalize, an awareness of problems, and the ability to use one's intellectual faculties. Group size ranges from eight to ten members, with a circular seating arrangement. The techniques used in the group are:

1. Isolating and defining the problem through open discussion, role playing, and exercises in communicating and establishing relationships.
2. Gathering information about the defined problem through open discussion.
3. Exploring methods to solve the problem, open discussion, and role playing. Feedback from group members can offer possible solutions. A problem always has at least four or five solutions.
4. Trying out the selected method. The participant must try to implement the selected method. This can be done by assigning the task to be completed by the next meeting.
5. Evaluating whether or not the selected method solved the problem in a reasonably satisfactory way.

An example of the problem-solving process is given in Chapter Two.

REALITY ORIENTATION

Reality orientation is a way to improve the quality of care for clients who are confused, or, more specifically, disoriented to time, place, things, and person. Causes for the impairment vary and may include cerebral deficit resulting from arteriosclerosis, head injury, stroke, sensory deprivation, overmedication, and drug and alcohol use. Long-term, chronic, mentally ill clients exhibiting disorientation have also been shown to benefit from reality orientation (Browne and Retter, 1972:139).

To be effective, reality orientation must be followed through on a 24-hour a day basis. Consequently, it involves all health providers. The health provider's total involvement makes success possible.

The techniques are simple and can be learned by any health provider who has demonstrated skill and patience in working with confused clients. "Reality orientation should not be confused with Reality Therapy (Glasser, 1965), which is conducted under the direction of a psychiatrist or other professional specifically trained in the theory and technique of Reality Therapy" (Taulbee, 1978:214).

Reality orientation begins immediately upon arising. When clients are awakened, they are addressed by name and oriented to time and day and what time breakfast will be served. The clients continue to be addressed by name throughout the day and are patiently reoriented to all aspects of care and scheduling during the day, evening, and night shifts. Use of the reality board, which has become an established part of most units with confused clients, is a helpful tool for the client as he struggles to remember information, such as where he is, the day of the week, date, and year. Additional information, such as the weather, next holiday, and next meal, are usually also included. Health providers must immediately reward current responses with verbal praise, a touch, or a smile, both on the unit and during group sessions.

Planned group sessions are held daily for 30 minutes, preferably at the same time each day. It is important that group sessions be held in the same room each time to provide consistency. The room itself must be pleasant, with plenty of light and table space. A basic group is limited to three or four very confused clients.

Ideally, the group has both a leader and a co-leader. Reality materials, such as a chalk board, felt board, large clock, and calendar, are essential props. Additional materials, such as jigsaw puzzles, maps, adult picture books, plastic fruit, vegetables, and flowers can be obtained from thrift stores. The use of these materials is limited only by the imagination. One way is to have clients associate an object with its name, which appears in large letters, such as an apple to the word APPLE.

At the beginning of each session, the client should review information already on the chalk board, such as the following (Lee, 1976:35):

The place is _____

The time is _____

The day of the week is _____

The date is _____

The weather is _____

The next holiday is _____

The next meal is _____

When the clients learn the simple information offered in the basic group, they are moved into the advanced group made up of eight to ten members. Memory games that are not too difficult—a sixth grade level is suggested—are excellent for stimulating recall and concentration. A somewhat more advanced version of the questions asked in the basic group is also useful. The group content should be varied enough so as not to become boring, but not so much as to be confusing. The advanced group sessions can also include grooming, physical exercise, and sensory training.

A trial period of two months is necessary to evaluate participants' progress. If at the end of that time the client shows no progress, it is best to discontinue his involvement in group sessions for the time being. The client can be readmitted to the group at a later date. Both groups must be evaluated monthly and changes made when indicated. The attitude of the leader and all health providers is most important to attaining the desired goals. Clients must not be embarrassed or singled out because of their confusion. Directions must be given in simple, short sentences and delivered in clear, distinct tones on an adult level. Information must be repeated as often as necessary. Clients need extra time for response, and the leader's expectant manner supports this expectation. Consistency in the routine, once it is established, is essential.

REMOTIVATION GROUP

"Remotivation therapy (RT) is a group technique for stimulating and revitalizing individuals who are no longer interested and involved in either the present or the future. This technique is essentially a structured program of discussion based on reality that uses objective materials to which individuals are encouraged to respond" (Dennis, 1978:219).

A remotivation group should not have more than 15 members. They should be willing to participate in a rather structured format. According to the Remotivation Technique Manual (Robinson), a total of 12 sessions is held, each session meeting once or twice a week for 30 minutes to an hour. Each session consists of five basic steps that all relate to one specific topic.

1. "Climate of acceptance," which includes introductions and getting acquainted (p. 7).

2. "Bridge to reality," which involves one of the members in reading an article or poem aloud (p. 7).

3. "Sharing the world we live in," which focuses on developing the topic through questions, visual aids, and props (p. 8).

4. "An appreciation of the work of the world," which encourages the members of the group to think about work in relation to themselves (p. 9).

5. "Climate of appreciation," which includes thanking the group for coming and planning for the next session (p. 9).

At the end of the 12 sessions, 12 different topics will have been discussed. Around the seventh session, the leader should remind the group that they are over halfway through and have only five more sessions. Remotivation therapy also includes techniques of sensory stimulation, reminiscing, and reality orientation.

EXAMPLE OF A REMOTIVATION SESSION

The topic for the session is the "Potato."

1. Step One. The members introduce themselves to one another. The leader comments on positive aspects of the members' appearance and dress.

2. Step Two. One of the group members is asked to read the rhyme, "One Potato, Two Potato, Three potato, Four."

3. Step Three. The leader asks the members of the group if they know how a potato grows. As members discuss a potato's growth, a real potato is passed around the group. Members are asked to describe the various kinds of potatoes. While this is going on, one member is asked to pass a dish of potato chips around the circle.

4. Step Four. A discussion begins about the work involved in preparing potatoes, from the garden to the market. Members are asked if they have ever been involved in similar work activity.

5. Step Five. The leader thanks group members for attending, and together they plan the topic for the next session, which they decide will be an animal, namely, the pig.

REMINISCENT GROUP

A reminiscent group utilizes the strengths and wisdom of the aged and in so doing gives members an opportunity to express themselves and develop a feeling of belongingness. Reminiscing also provides memory stimulation, an increased sense of one's identity, socialization, recreation, and self-actualization (Ebersole, 1978:237–243). Sometimes older persons, who in their mid-life had really developed their creative ability, have been unable to continue at this level because of confinement to their home or a facility. It is possible that through group reminiscing this level of human need can be met, and the individual can once again use his creative talents.

Life review therapy, which was developed by Butler, involves reminiscing as a way of understanding and accepting the meaning of one's life (Butler, 1963:65–76). It is seen as psychotherapy for the elderly, since it focuses on surveying old conflicts with reintegration.

The membership of a reminiscent group should be limited to five or six clients. Usually these groups are held for about ten sessions, each one hour in length. It is important that the group leader approach each potential group member individually and invite that person to attend meetings to talk about the past. The leader must express interest in learning about each member's history. Also, each member must be told who the other members will be, since each person must be free to make his own decision about attending (Huber, Miller, 1984:84–85). It is helpful to gather in the same place, at the same time each week.

Group meetings should begin with introductions. Sometimes relaxation exercises, music, and snacks are ways of increasing verbal responsiveness. Another way to begin reminiscing is to have the members locate their birthplace on a map and then tell whatever they can remember about it (Ebersole, 1978:249). Other topics that will evoke memories include members' hobbies, jobs, celebration of certain holidays, favorite bands, singers, radio shows, movie stars, cars, and inventions. Props, such as bright visual aids, selected picture books, old newspapers, and old tools or farm equipment, can stimulate conversation (McMordie and Blom, 1979:165). Termination of a reminiscent group can sometimes be difficult because of the many personal memories that have been shared. "The resolution of the pain of termination lies in the concept of reminiscence. Remembering is the means for holding on and letting go" (Ebersole, 1978:251).

Karen Kruschke, R.N., in an article entitled "Who Determines What Is Real?" states that "for the elderly, reality—and happiness—often lives in their memories." In that article, she tells the story of a disoriented 85-year-old man, formerly a farmer, who was placed in a nursing home. After he became oriented to his surroundings, he questioned why everything had to be real and true. He went on to say, "I'll tell you what's really the truth. I want to die. I want to be with my wife. I hate it when you people won't leave me alone with my memories. I loved life then . . . those were the only days that counted. I know I can't have my cows here, but can't I pretend sometimes? Is that so wrong?" Ebersole, in a presentation on Reminiscence and Aging at the 22nd Annual Meeting of the Western Gerontological Society mentioned that psychologist Robert Kastenbaum "thinks the older person avoids thoughts of the future because he has so little of it left and that little holds more unpleasant prospects than pleasant ones" (Nathanson and Stunkel, 1976:259).

SENSORY STIMULATION GROUP

Sensory stimulation is a very important part of infant development and is a natural part of the care that a young child receives. Studies, especially those by René Spitz, have demonstrated the effects that sensory and emotional deprivation have on the infant's development (Spitz, 1965:280).

Throughout the life cycle, sensory stimulation continues to be a significant aspect of the growth process. However, most individuals are able to meet this need because they participate in many activities in the outside world. It is the individual who is unable to move about in the outside world due to illness or age who can experience sensory deprivation and requires sensory stimulation.

A sensory stimulation group should be small, no more than six members. They should be seated in a tight circle so that their knees or arms are close to the person on each side, and the leader can easily reach out and touch the members without getting out of his chair. The leader needs to relate to the group members with warmth and supportiveness, explaining that the purpose of the group is to stimulate their senses. Focusing on one sense during a session, which is about 30 minutes in length, will maximize the stimulation in one area.

Props that can be used for sensory stimulation include:

1. **Sight props.** Clocks, calendars, bright colors, pictures, mirrors, windows, houseplants, flowers.
2. **Sound props.** Meaningful conversation, singing, music, children's voices; choices of radio, stereo or T.V., piano, tambourine.
3. **Touch props.** Back rub, massage, holding hands, feeling different textures. A bag with pieces of various materials, such as velvet, fur, burlap, silk, and corduroy, can be passed around the group. With eyes closed, each member puts his hand into the bag and tries to identify the materials.
4. **Smell props.** Varied and appetizing foods, perfume and cologne, powder,

flowers, and spices. One sensory training program used the spices of tea, tobacco, cinnamon, and almond extract. Each person in the group would smell each item, then tell the group what he thought the item was. Praise was given for the correct answer; if the answer was incorrect, the individual would smell the item again while repeating its name, and then receive reinforcement for saying it correctly (Heidell, 1972:40).

5. **Taste props.** Varied and appetizing foods, especially fresh fruits, good oral hygiene, varied fluids. Heidell, in her sensory training program, used Lifesavers and asked the members of the group to relate the color of the Lifesaver to the flavor (Heidell, 1972:40).

6. **Internal stimulation props.** Exercise, walking, stretching, movement therapy, relaxation therapy, dancing.

Correcting sensory deprivation is a fundamental responsibility of the health provider (Burnside, 1978:214). By intervening with sensory exercises, the provider can retard the progression of deterioration in the elderly client.

EDUCATION GROUP

The education group is based on the philosophy that the client should be "knowledgeable about his illness and should be active in his treatment plan, thus enabling him to become involved with health maintenance and disease prevention" (Consumer Health Education Brochure).

It is important that the education group be run as a school; therefore, instead of the staff/client relationship, there is a teacher/student relationship. In the education group, the client is taught the skills he needs to improve his functioning in society.

There are different ways of setting up the education group, but some basic commonalities are evident in all of the approaches. First, the education approach includes classes with specific curriculum for which clients register. Pretests and post-tests are given, and sometimes the classes are offered on a semester basis. Depending on the staff's expertise, many can be involved, along with volunteer students from a local college or university and community agencies, such as the Red Cross and telephone company. Classes are usually small, no more than 10 persons. Subjects taught can run the gamut from personal care through daily living skills, to leisure time activities, to classes relevant to community involvement (Spiegler, 1977:224). In the "Consumer Health Education" program, entitled "School of Living," at Greystone Park Psychiatric Hospital, a course was taught on human behavior. Course topics included communication and awareness, loneliness, anger, self-appraisal, love and human communication, and human sexuality (Sclafani, 1976:948).

Usually a class on medication is an important area that is covered in an education program, since remaining on medication after discharge is a problem for many persons who have psychiatric problems. At the Community Training Center, established at the Palo Alto (California) Veterans Administration Hospital in 1970, a "Humor Class" was offered, since it was felt that the lack of a sense of humor was a common behavioral deficit. This class consisted of listening to comedy records, telling funny stories, writing limericks, reading jokes, and watching comedy shows on television (Spiegler, 1977:224). Through education groups/classes, independent strengths, self-esteem, and social enlightenment are fostered among groups of people who happen to be clients.

CLIENT GOVERNMENT

Client government can be viewed as a therapeutic intervention because the client participates in decision-making and the responsibility that goes with it. The structure varies according to the needs of the facility, but in most cases the clients and health provider meet together once or twice a week to deal with day-to-day problems. Client government is based on some key ideas, such as (1) having clients make and enforce most of the unit rules; (2) taking care of most routine unit tasks; and (3) solving many of the problems of unit-living by themselves. Some of the problems dealt with by the client government include other client's acting-out behavior, the unit's cleanliness, use of television, client complaints, ideas on remodeling the unit, and social activities.

The health provider's philosophy and the policy of the facility determine if client government will be utilized or permitted in the facility. If the philosophy is based on the idea that "the health providers know best," it will be difficult to accept suggestions and decisions based on client government. If the health provider sees himself as playing a supportive role, rather than as the victim of client government, there is a good chance that it can work. First of all, the health provider must realize that the provider does not sit by providing no input while the clients run the unit. Instead, the health provider offers his ideas on the issues being discussed and, as in a democratic situation, abides by the group's decisions. The constitution and by-laws of the client government need to state what responsibilities belong to the clients, so that legal issues, such as medications and passes, are not confused with the activities of daily living issues. The health provider may be surprised to discover that some clients resent being a part of the decision-making process, since this is one of the reasons for leaving their outside living situation.

Historically, clients have depended on the health provider to provide ideas and activities for them and have been upset when such resources were inadequate or uninteresting. Much of the inactivity and boredom that clients complain about can be dealt with directly through client government as clients assume more responsibility for themselves. Client government that is supported by the health provider offers a way for clients to learn how health providers formulate their decisions and to provide input into the decisions as well. It is also a way for clients to respond to one another's needs. Through group pressure, clients can provide support and assistance in controlling inappropriate behavior. Client government on the positive side is one way of supporting the independence that health providers verbally encourage for their clientele and of giving the client some sense of control over his own life.

REFERENCES

Backer, B., Dubbert, P., and Eisenman, E., 1978. Psychiatric/Mental Health Nursing: Contemporary Readings. New York, D. Van Nostrand Company.

Berger, M., 1977. Working With People Called Patients. New York, Brunner/Mazel, Publishers.

Burnside, I., 1978. Working With The Elderly: Group Process And Techniques. North Scituate, MA, Duxbury Press.

Butler, R., 1963. The life review: An interpretation of reminiscence in the aged. Psychiatry, Vol. 26, pp. 65–76.

Consumer Health Education Brochure. Greystone, N.J., Greystone Park Psychiatric Hospital.

Cordero, J., n.d. Reminiscing: A Meaningful Activity for the Elderly. Madison, WI, Restorative Care Associates, Inc.

Dennis, H., 1978. Remotivation therapy groups. In Burnside, I. (ed): Working With The Elderly: Group Process And Techniques. North Scituate, MA, Duxbury Press.

Dunlap, L., 1978. Conducting a Therapeutic Community. In Mental Health Concepts Applied to Nursing. New York, John Wiley & Sons.

Ebersole, P., 1978. Establishing Reminiscing Groups. In Burnside, I. (ed): Working With The Elderly: Group Process and Techniques. North Scituate, MA, Duxbury Press.

A Theoretical Approach to the Use of Reminiscence. In Burnside, I. (ed): Working With The Elderly: Group Process And Techniques. North Scituate, MA, Duxbury Press.

Folsom, J.C., 1968. Reality orientation for the elderly mental patient. J Geriatr Psychiatry, Vol. 1, p. 291.

Franclemont, J., and Sclafani, M., 1978. Self-medication program for the emotionally ill. J Psychosoc Nurs Ment Health Serv, January, pp. 15–17.

Goble, F., 1970. The Third Force. The Psychology of Abraham Maslow. New York, Grossman Publishers.

Goldstein, A., Sprafkin, R., and Gershaw, N., 1976. Skill Training For Community Living. Elmsford, N.Y., Pergamon Press, Inc. (37 basic skill audio tapes.)

Hahn, J., and Burns, K., 1973. Mrs. Richards, a rabbit, and remotivation. Am J Nurs, February, pp. 302–305.

Heidell, B., 1972. Sensory training puts patients 'in touch'. Modern Nurs Home, Vol. 28, June, pp. 39–43.

Howe, J., Dickason, E., Jones, D., and Snider, M., 1984. The Handbook of Nursing. New York, John Wiley & Sons.

Huber, K., and Miller, P., 1984. Reminisce with the elderly—Do it! Geriatr Nurs, March/April, pp. 84–87.

King, K., 1982. Reminiscing psychotherapy with aging people. J Psychosoc Nurs Ment Health Serv, February, pp. 21–25.

Kruschke, K., 1983. Who Determines What Is Real? Family Weekly, The Milwaukee Journal, July 3, pp. 14–15.

Lee, R., 1976. Reality Orientation: Restoring the Senile to Life. J Pract Nurs, January, pp. 28–37.

McMordie, W., and Blom, S., 1979. Life review therapy: Psychotherapy for the elderly. Perspect Psychiatr Care, Vol. 28, No. 4, pp. 162–166.

Robinson, A., n.d. Remotivation Technique. American Psychiatric Association Mental Hospital Service and the Smith Kline and French Laboratories Project.

Scarbrough, D., 1974. Reality orientation: A new approach to an old problem. Nursing '74. November, pp. 12–13.

Scheideman, J., 1976. Remotivation: Involvement without labels. J Psychosoc Nurs Ment Health Serv, July, pp. 41–42.

Sclafani, M., 1977. Medication classes for the emotionally ill. J Psychosoc Nurs Ment Health Serv, April, pp. 13–16.

Sclafani, M., 1976. School for psychiatric patients. Am J Nurs, June, pp. 948–949.

Spiegler, M., and Agigian, H., 1977. The Community Training Center. An Educational–Behavioral–Social Systems Model for Rehabilitating Psychiatric Patients. New York, Brunner/Mazel, Publishers.

Spiegler, M., 1977. School days—Creditable treatment. Psychiatr Q, Vol. 49, No. 3, pp. 221–229.

Spitz, R., 1965. The First Year of Life: A Psychoanalytic Study of Normal and Deviant Development of Object Relations. New York, International Press, Inc.

Taulbee, L., 1978. Reality orientation: A therapeutic group activity for elderly persons. In Burnside, I. (ed): Working With The Elderly: Group Process and Techniques. North Scituate, MA, Duxbury Press.

Trotter, R., 1972. Reality orientation. Sci News, December 23, p. 411.

Wilson, H., and Kneisl, C., 1979. Psychiatric Nursing. Menlo Park, CA, Addison-Wesley Publishing.

Nathanson, J., and Stunkel, E., 1976. Reminiscence and Aging. In Aging in the Tricentennium: Assuming a Shared Responsibility. San Francisco, The Proceedings of the 22nd Annual Meeting of the Western Gerontological Society.

ESSENCE OF STAYING ALIVE AS A HEALTH PROVIDER— STRESS MANAGEMENT

LEARNING OBJECTIVES—Upon completing this chapter, the reader will be able to:

1. Discuss two ways that client care can produce stress for the health provider.

2. Differentiate between an empathic and sympathetic response to the client.

3. Explain what is meant by Thomas' quote regarding work stress.

4. Describe how to deal with a person who constantly makes personal attacks.

5. List two positive reasons for evaluating one's own performance daily.

6. Give two suggestions for organizing a hectic day.

7. Identify three functions accomplished with humor in the work setting.

8. List six ways of relieving personal stress.

The health provider must learn to take care of himself so that he can, in turn, use himself more effectively in relating to the emotionally disturbed client. In taking care of himself positively, he serves as a desirable role model for both co-workers and client. Without a doubt, client care can produce stress for the health provider. Clients can be demanding and press for magically dramatic solutions to their problems. Regressive behavior often peaks more severely in the mentally ill client than in the physically ill client. Often, client needs are expressed indirectly, through irritability or criticism of the health provider's performance. In addition, client problems and behaviors can unleash unresolved personal problems that the health provider has not come to terms with. For example, client problems can look very much like those being experienced by family members or friends; sometimes the health provider knew the client in happier times. Emotional illness, with its complexities, involves the entire client, including his physical health, which is often at stake. The client may not respond to treatment and may continue to deteriorate. Life and death issues may be at stake. Lack of cooperation by the client and his family may cause the health provider to feel angry and frustrated. The provider may be tempted to blame the client for causing him to feel helpless and for the client's lack of improvement. Clients may challenge the care they're receiving and the knowledge base of involved staff. Family members may call continuously because of concern, lack of understanding, and feelings of helplessness.

Differentiating between feelings of empathy and sympathy in regard to the client is a major consideration in preventing burnout. Empathy is a respectful, detached concern; the provider understands what the client is experiencing but does not experience the emotion with him. Sympathy, on the other hand, leaves the provider vulnerable to identifying with the client and experiencing the emotion along with the client. The provider is no longer in control of the situation and has limited long-range value to the client; thus, a long-term sympathetic response is very stressful. What started out as a caring relationship becomes detrimental to the client and provider because of over-involvement.

One can deal with the stress of work as suggested by Thomas in the following statements: ". . . the only question, I am inclined to turn aside as being impossible to respond to happens to be the one most often raised these days, not just by my biologist friends but by everyone; the question about stress, how to avoid stress, prevent stress, allay stress. I refuse to have anything to do with this matter, having made up my mind, from everything I have read or heard about it in recent years, that what people mean by stress is simply the condition of being human, and I will not recommend any meddling with it, by medicine or any other profession," (1983:71). He has a point! As noted earlier in the book, it is not the event, but rather one's reaction to it that determines the amount of stress experienced.

Viktor Frankl proclaims, "Change your attitude if you can't change the situation" (Frankl, 1984: Workshop, "Man's Search for Meaning"). He should know. He lived through grim conditions in concentration camps yet continued his personal growth within those circumstances, going on to become one of the most renowned psychiatrists in the world. He further cautions against aiming at success. "Aim at what your conscience wants you to do. Each man knows in his heart what his assignment in life is. Success will follow you. Like happiness, the more you aim, the more you miss. Give yourself to a cause" (Frankl: Workshop, "Man's Search for Meaning"). Life is an adventure, and, as pointed out in Isaiah, 14:24, "Surely as I think so shall it come to pass." In other words, stop comparing yourself to others and running yourself down. As long as you thwart your own self-image, it will be difficult to deal with others in a positive way. Think "I can" and "I will." Unless limited in a physical way, most of the "I can't" statements really mean, "I won't." In working with emotionally ill clients, the provider is the major tool, and the provider's personality is a reflection of his attitudes. It is interesting to note that as one gives up criticizing, experiencing guilt, and harshly judging oneself, others seem friendlier, too. Mutual trust of the co-worker begins with the provider. This does not mean the provider won't be hurt occasionally by those who violate this trust. However, honesty and a willingness to deal directly with difficult people often pays off. Bramson (1984:46–47) suggests the following basic rules for dealing with those who attack you: (1) Stand up for yourself—otherwise, you'll be ignored. (2) Don't worry about being rude—when the other person is interrupting, tell him, then keep on talking. (3) Get the difficult person to sit down—most people are less aggressive when sitting down. (4) Speak from your point of view; use I-centered statements. (5) Avoid an all-out fight. Your purpose is to function more effectively. (6) Be ready to be friendly. Once you have stood up to the difficult person, the offer is usually genuine.

Developing a detached way of evaluating daily personal performance is also helpful. Waiting for the boss to notice rarely works; perhaps he will notice only what is missing. However, a detached, daily evaluation of self leaves the health provider free to give himself credit for what he has done well and alerts him to areas that need more study and practice. The health provider should not harbor hard feelings because the boss failed to meet his expectations. The health provider himself is his most important boss. He should not worry about what others think.

Many of the suggestions for dealing with daily events in the work world emphasize time management. It pays to come in a few minutes early and make several lists: (1) Must do, (2) Nice to do, and (3) Can wait. The lists can be revised as the day progresses. Don't be afraid to delegate or ask for help. Pace yourself, and beware of squeezing in any items from the "Nice to do" list until all the "Must do" items are completed. Remember also to say "No" to requests that are not "Must do's" in an emergency-packed day. Beware also of the chronic complainers and the temptation to do their work just to quiet them down. Brief periods of relaxation on a busy day are "Must do's." Consider some of the brief relaxation techniques described in Chapter 10. The techniques range from one to ten minutes or more; one can even be done while walking down the hall, while in the bathroom, or while on a break.

The essence of staying alive as a health provider, however, is in maintaining a sense of humor. Freud supported it. What additional endorsement is needed? Humor in the work setting accomplishes three functions according to Robinson (1977:40). It communicates important messages, promotes social relationships, diminishes the discomforts, and manages "delicate" situations that occur in this setting. Humor is also an equalizer among health providers and, in many instances, between client and health provider. Robinson provides the following example of this (1977:44): A mental health center attempted to foster a blurring of roles by asking health providers to wear street clothes rather than uniforms. The providers were still obliged to wear name tags identifying their title, which continued to set them apart. The controversy finally ended when a client appeared one morning wearing a name tag that read, Mary Smith, N.U.T.! Point made; problem solved! In another example, a physician client was expected to produce a urine specimen each morning. The first morning the health provider entered his room and announced, "It's time for our specimen." The second morning, the specimen container was already filled. When the health provider announced, "I've come for our specimen," the client picked up the container, drank half of it, and handed it to the provider, saying, "Here's your half of our specimen." Shocked, the provider retreated only to discover that the client had substituted his morning juice for the real thing! He had accomplished all three functions of humor with one quick drink.

One final note. There is life after clients. The health provider's private life, which provides for *self-care,* sets a positive example for both clients and peers. Ways to take care of oneself are limited only by one's imagination. The following additional suggestions range from humorous to serious. The provider is invited to sit back, relax, and let his imagination flow. For convenience, the suggestions have been categorized as personal, professional, and both.

PERSONAL	**PROFESSIONAL**
1. Give your full attention to what is happening at the moment. When you are with your family members, concentrate on what is going on with them, rather than what went on at work that day.	1. Teach yourself to worry only when the situation is at hand. Your supervisor has sent a message that she wants to see you next Friday. Consciously make the decision to postpone concern about this meeting until Friday.
2. Realize that some ongoing problems can never be fully resolved, such as money, sex, family, and aging.	2. Focus on your area of responsibility, and channel energy into that area. As a health provider, you have an assigned number of clients; direct your energies toward their care.
3. Do the things that you have been postponing. For example, take a walk in the woods; get in touch with an old friend.	3. Arrange for vacation periods rather than a single day off here and there.
4. Plan for a quiet time in your day that will give you a sense of peace and tranquility. Drift off into a quiet state with silence, music, or a beautiful scene.	4. Rotate work assignments or vary tasks within an assignment.
5. Select activities outside the work setting that are different from the tasks at work. If work demands heavy mental concentration, do something physical, and vice versa.	5. Use your travel time from work to home as a bridge to a relaxing evening. Plan some small, special reward for the evening, such as calling a friend, or taking a walk.
6. Maintain a focus on the positive aspects of what is going on at the time. See your glass as half-full, rather than as half-empty.	6. Start a support group among your colleagues— not to gripe, but to share ways of coping.
7. Attempt to space major life events when possible, such as a new job, starting school, moving, marriage.	7. Make a list of all the things you don't like about your job; put the list away for a week, then rewrite the list. Continue to rewrite your list weekly, and the real problems will begin to emerge.
8. Tune into the body signal system, especially migratory aches and pains, such as headaches, backaches, constant fatigue, irritability, sleeping problems.	8. When facing a situation that is threatening to you, imagine the other people involved as being naked. It really works!

Table continues on following page.

PERSONAL

9. If hungry when upset, limit your diet to light foods that are easily digested.
10. Choose a friend who supports your strengths.
11. Breathe slowly, and pay attention to the air going in and out of your nostrils.
12. Lie on the floor with feet up on a chair and a cool wash cloth on your face; think of the most peaceful scene you can imagine.
13. Enlarge your world by doing things for others outside the work setting, such as volunteer work.
14. Identify positive outlets that have worked for you before in dealing with your emotional discomfort, such as dancing, card games, needlepoint, volleyball.
15. Balance food intake with physical activity.
16. Take a walk instead of a martini!
17. Avoid self-medication with alcohol and drugs.
18. Rehearse or reconstruct in your mind a familiar humorous story.
19. Divide large projects into a series of small actions with beginnings and endings, such as cleaning one room thoroughly each week, rather than the whole house.
20. Give in occasionally, even if you are right. If you yield once in awhile, you'll find that others will too.
21. Develop and maintain social contacts.
22. Go into a room, close the door, and cry or scream; then take 10 minutes to do what is most relaxing.
23. Schedule time for relaxation so that work and play are balanced.
24. Get up early enough to prepare a good breakfast for the day.
25. Loaf a little; nap a little. Everybody needs "do-nothing" time.
26. Focus on the process of a project, rather than the final result. This helps one gain satisfaction from what he is doing, regardless of the problems encountered along the way. At Christmastime, focus on all of the preparations—baking, decorating, purchasing gifts—rather than concentrating on whether or not everything will be done by Christmas.
27. Develop leisure activities that can be continued throughout the life span.
28. Ask a friend to give you a massage.
29. Limit intake of fats, sugar, salt, additives, and caffeine. Make food choices within the four basic food groups: fruits and vegetables; milk and milk products; cereals and breads; meat, fish, dried peas and beans.
30. Pull the drapes, lock the door, strip, put on the music you enjoy, and dance to your heart's content!
31. Get enough sleep and rest.
32. Pause when you enter a room, and survey the situation before plunging in.
33. Get involved in an organized physical activity, such as swimming, jazzercise, baseball, tennis.
34. Write a letter to the person with whom you are

PROFESSIONAL

9. Resolve to discuss nonwork-related topics during breaks and mealtime.
10. Allow yourself time to change roles—from worker to family member; from student to child role. Give yourself an "unwinding time."

BOTH

1. Grieve your past losses—death, divorce, major surgery, loss of a job—and then go on with living.
2. Re-evaluate goals to be sure they are realistic and attainable. If you do not accomplish all that you had planned for the day, it is possible your plans were unrealistic.
3. Decide what is important, and then request it. Persons are not mind readers. If you need additional help, request it. You may not get it, but at least you asked for it!
4. Stay away from negative people. Negativism can be contagious.
5. At the end of the day, congratulate yourself on at least one positive accomplishment for the day.
6. When all the "cards seem down," remind yourself that there is only one way to go, and that is *up*!
7. There is always more than one way to solve a problem. Use your imagination to consider all possible solutions.
8. After a bad day, relax in a hot shower and sing to your heart's content. No one can hear you if the shower is running hard enough.
9. Cultivate a sense of humor. Exaggerate the distressing situation to the point that it is ridiculous or view the entire event as a cartoon and get in touch with some of the ridiculousness of what upset you.
10. Ask yourself the question, "Will what now seems to be an overwhelming problem still be that significant 10 years from now?"
11. Give yourself permission to make mistakes. Remind yourself that "this is the first time that I am this age, facing the exact situation; so I am doing the best I can."
12. Make a list of unresolved problems and tasks. Just the act of getting them out of your head and onto paper is a way of "parking" them for the next day.
13. If you must complain, be prepared to offer an alternative solution and be willing to help in its implementation.
14. Trust yourself to make decisions about your own life; after all, you know yourself better than anyone else does. By trusting yourself, others will respect and trust you.
15. Limit your "poor me" time. Decide on the amount of time you need to feel sorry for yourself; allow yourself to experience the feeling, then let go of it.
16. Accept responsibility for your failure; admit that you "goofed." The important question is, "What are you going to do about it?"

PERSONAL

upset, saying just how you feel; then tear it up.

35. Greet or meet one new person every day; work at this.

36. Force yourself to do something for someone in need when you feel "down in the dumps."

37. Keep a diary of your activities to help identify the pattern of stress in your life.

38. Be aware of when you normally awake, then get up and start your day. Don't try to go back to sleep.

39. If it feels too risky to confront a person directly, *imagine* him in a chair in front of you; tell him exactly what you want to tell him, sparing no detail.

40. Imagine you can have anything in the world, except that it cannot be related to money. For what you want, you must give up something in return.

41. Plan for 20 minutes of uninterrupted quiet once or twice a day, preferably not after eating. After relaxing your body, say aloud a word with a soft sound, such as calm or love. Repeat the word until you hear your unspoken voice; sit quietly hearing the mental repetition of the word. If other thoughts enter in, guide your attention back to the word.

42. Go window shopping or shopping, as the budget allows.

43. Use self-massage to touch away tension in the areas where you feel pressure.

44. Scrub the floor, clean the house, mow the lawn, bake bread, cut firewood; these are all constructive, physical outlets for relieving pent-up feelings.

45. Settle your arguments before going to bed at night.

46. A glass of warm milk before bedtime provides a natural sedative for sleep.

47. If you are struggling with a problem for which you have no solution, tell yourself before you go to sleep at night that you will have an answer to the problem when you awaken.

48. Read a sad book, go to a sad movie, or watch a sad T.V. show, and let yourself cry.

49. Seek professional counseling.

BOTH

17. Get your fears and worries out in the open. Find someone you respect and trust and air your feelings, no matter how absurd they are.

18. Own your own feelings. If you are angry with someone, tell him how you feel, using "I" messages instead of blaming the person for your feelings.

19. Imagine having less discomfort three months from now than you have at this time.

20. Remember that rejection of your values is not a rejection of you.

21. Become the solution rather than part of the problem.

22. Refuse to feel embarrassed. After all, to err is human.

23. Call what you are experiencing by its real name. If you are angry, say that you are angry. Don't use terms such as guilty, irritable, upset.

24. Focus on your successes rather than your failures. You cannot help everyone.

25. Keep time in perspective. Do not expect results right away.

26. Allow others to own their problems and to be responsible for their behavior.

27. Learn to accept help. Life is a balance of giving and taking.

28. Change activities when you feel yourself tensing up.

29. Rehearse in advance what you are going to say in a situation that you anticipate as being stressful.

30. Repeat calming statements to yourself, such as, "Now take it easy; I can handle it."

31. Differentiate between what can be changed and what cannot be changed, and use your energies accordingly.

32. Look for one positive point in the person you are angry with, and share that positive attribute with the individual.

33. If you feel trapped in your situation, ask yourself if you want to get out. If the answer is yes, do it; if the answer is no, look for ways to change your daily work environment.

34. Fantasize taking a vacation and having a very good time.

35. Plan a time for voicing your complaints; stick to your schedule. Avoid airing your grievances at other times.

36. Identify your time span for concentration. Consciously time yourself, and you will see a pattern emerge. Take brief breaks after your periods of concentration, and your work efficiency will improve.

37. Utilize your energies to find solutions to your problems rather than to try to figure out why you feel the way you do. Usually the reason is obvious anyway.

38. If a problem seems impossible, put it on the shelf for awhile. When you return, you'll have a fresh perspective.

39. Listen to what the other person is saying to you. Check out what you are hearing to be sure you understand.

REFERENCES

Bramson, R., 1984. Assertive techniques for handling difficult people. Nurs Life, July/August, pp. 46–49.

Frankl, V., 1984. Man's Search For Meaning, Workshop, Mount Mary College, Milwaukee, WI.

Hamilton, J., 1984. Effective ways to relieve stress. Nurs Life, July/August, pp. 24–27

Robinson, V., 1977. Humor and the Health Professions. Thorofare, NJ, Charles Slack, Inc.

Thomas, L., 1983. Late Night Thoughts on Listening to Mahler's Ninth Symphony. New York, Viking Press.

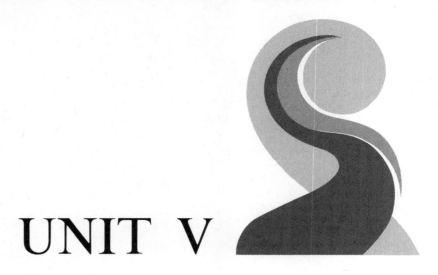

UNIT V

INTERVENTIONS TO MEET SPECIFIC NEEDS

PSYCHOPHARMACOLOGY AND OTHER PHYSICAL/ MEDICAL THERAPIES

LEARNING OBJECTIVES—Upon completing this chapter, the reader will be able to:

1.   Describe the four classifications of psychotherapeutic medications.

2.   List three physical/medical therapies used prior to the introduction of psycho-therapeutic medications.

PSYCHOPHARMACOLOGY*

Psychopharmacology is the study of medications that are used to reduce and control symptoms of emotional disturbances. They do not "cure" the illness but rather decrease symptoms so that the client can function more effectively and, in some instances, be more amenable to other therapies.

Among the many theories regarding mental illness is one that attributes it to biochemical changes in the brain. Neurotransmitter substances (e.g., dopamine) are needed to transmit messages at the synapse, a fluid-filled space between the neurons. When the impulse (message) arrives at the synapse, it triggers the release of a chemical called a neurotransmitter. "At no point does one of the neurons touch each other; signals are passed spark gap fashion. At each firing one nerve chemically communicates with another" (Ratcliff, 1983:13). A synapse is diagrammed in Figure 13–1.

Evidence indicates, for example, that severe depression may result from a decrease in neurotransmitters, while an increase in these substances may produce a manic state. The prescribed medications attack the neurotransmitter substance, the goal being to correct the imbalance. Some medications block the neurotransmitter, some increase it, and some limit the amount of neurotransmitter that is released.

It is easier to think of these medications according to their classification, rather than as individual drugs. All medications within a class have essentially the same action, range of side effects, and specific considerations for the health provider. In addition, all medications that belong to a classification produce about an equal degree of improvement. However, one medication within the classification may work for a client when another from the same classification has been ineffective. Sometimes medications are chosen for a specific side effect. For example, a sedating side effect may be beneficial to the client who has been unable to sleep because of a manic episode, severe depression, or pathological suspiciousness. Within this framework, it becomes more convenient for the provider to

---

*This section was written with the assistance of Paul A. Schanen, R.Ph.

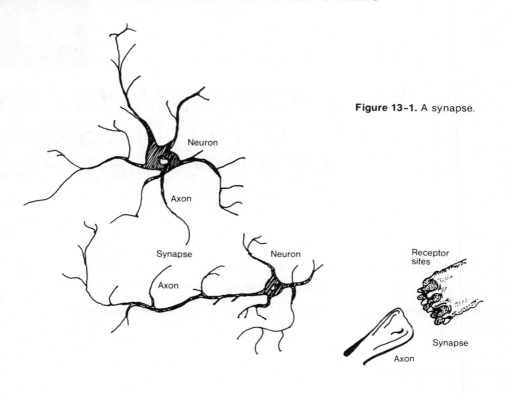

Figure 13-1. A synapse.

learn about similarities in each classification, fitting in individual variations in side effects should they occur. New medications within a classification are continually being developed. Since they are often structurally similar to the pre-existing drugs, the information just described is applicable to these new drugs as well.

The following four drug classifications will be discussed:
—Antipsychotic agents (major tranquilizers)
—Antianxiety agents (minor tranquilizers)
—Antidepressive agents (mood elevators)
—Antimanic agents

A list of common medications and their trade and generic names is included at the end of each classification.

ANTIPSYCHOTIC AGENTS

In the mid-1950s, a new drug that had been developed to deal with surgical shock was accidentally discovered to have powerful antipsychotic properties. The drug, chlorpromazine (Thorazine), changed the course of psychiatric care. Because chlorpromazine reduced psychotic symptomatology so dramatically, it became possible to negotiate a change from custodial client care to therapeutic programs that led to clients' discharge and their return to community living.

Although these medications were initially called major tranquilizers, the term tranquilizer does not describe the actual change that occurs in the client. Essentially, the client's behavior becomes more socially acceptable. "Target symptoms most likely to improve from the use of antipsychotic drugs include hyperactivity, combativeness, agitation, hostility, hallucinations, irritability, negativism, acute delusions, insomnia, poor self care and anorexia while there is less likely to be improvement in memory, orientation, apathy, withdrawal, retardation, insight and judgment" (Mason and Granacher, 1980:8).

Approximately one to five days of medication are necessary before a reduction in a client's acute psychotic symptoms is evident and his cooperation is obtained. About six weeks are necessary for total improvement.

Like the anxiety agents, antipsychotic medications have an additive effect when combined with other central nervous system (CNS) depressants, such as alcohol. This may become a concern when a client leaves on pass. It is unrealistic to think that a client who is used to consuming some alcohol will be willing to give it up entirely. He may instead decide to give up the medication. How the health provider deals with this issue will often determine the client's course of action. Always explain to the client that his medication has a long-term effect. Then suggest striking a balance, such as limiting his drinking to one glass of beer, wine, or sherry. Encourage the client to be aware of the effect of alcohol, and follow through with a discussion when he returns.

The antipsychotic medications as a group are safe. While dangerous side effects can occur, they are rare. Half of all side effects occur within the first week of therapy.

Sedation is one of the most common side effects, and, as with most side effects, the body develops a tolerance in a week or two. The client experiencing sedation does not initiate conversation or activity and tends to respond with one word answers. It is difficult for the client to participate in other aspects of treatment while experiencing this side effect.

Extrapyramidal side effects (EPS) include dystonia, akathisia, pseudoparkinsonism, and tardive dyskinesia. All of these side effects involve muscle control. The dystonias usually happen within 24 to 48 hours and are characterized by bizarre, involuntary, painful muscle contractions that usually involve the back, neck muscles, and mouth area. The symptoms are frightening and need prompt treatment with an antiparkinson agent. Akathisia, often described as motor restlessness, is more common in women. The behavior can often be differentiated from psychotic agitation by distracting the client with something of personal interest. If the behavior is part of the client's problem, he can generally be distracted. If the restlessness is due to akathisia, it will continue, regardless of the distraction attempts. Pseudoparkinsonism is drug-induced, and symptoms such as tremors, rigidity, masked facies, and shuffling gait are part of this syndrome. Antiparkinson agents, such as Cogentin, Artane, and Benadryl, relieve symptoms. Levadopa does not relieve drug-induced parkinsonism (Medical Letter, 1983:50). "Tardive dyskinesia is one of the most serious adverse effects of drugs used to treat schizophrenia; it usually occurs after prolonged therapy and sometimes persists for long periods or for life even after the drug is discontinued" (Medical Letter:50). So far no drugs have been identified as effective in treating tardive dyskinesia, which means late occurring dystonia. The condition involves bizarre movements of the lips, tongue, and cheek, such as lip smacking, sucking, and puckering. Sometimes the fingers, toes, or trunk become involved. The health provider is encouraged to check the client's tongue regularly for vermiform (wormlike) movements, which are often the first sign of tardive dyskinesia. Have the client open his mouth and keep his tongue on the floor of the mouth. Observe for the rolling, worm-like movement of the tongue.

Anticholinergic effects include dry mouth, dysphagia, postural hypotension, urinary hesitancy or retention, constipation, and anhidrosis. Many clients experience dry mouth. This is usually mild and transient. The client frequently describes the sensation as a mouth full of cotton. Rinsing the mouth or taking small sips of water is helpful. The mechanical action of chewing sugarless gum releases some saliva. Saliva-stimulating gum, such as Quench, is also known to be helpful (Greist and Jefferson, 1984:48). Sugared candy and gum is discouraged, since the lack of saliva promotes development of *Candida* (yeast) infection in the mouth. The risk of gum and tooth decay is also increased. Clients with dentures may benefit from using paste instead of a powder adhesive, since the powder is dependent on saliva to achieve the adhesive mix. Additional fluid between bites of food with adequate chewing time is essential during meals. Dysphagia, the inability to swallow, is potentially serious and may lead to choking or silent aspiration. It can often be identified at mealtime when the client lets liquids, such as milk, run out of his mouth. Solids, as a rule, are easier to swallow, but supervision is needed during meals. Postural or orthostatic hypotension means that the client experiences a sudden drop in blood pressure when he goes from a reclining to a standing position. Although a temporary symptom usually, it can result in injury and falls, especially among the elderly. Instruct the client to dangle his legs for a few minutes before getting up and to get up slowly. Elastic stockings may also be helpful during this time. Lying down for one-half hour after an intramuscular injection is recommended. However, if the client was agitated to begin with, chances are he will jump up. Be prepared to catch him! Should he black out, laying him down with his feet higher than the rest of his body will be helpful. As with all of the anticholinergic effects, poor hydration increases the hypotensive effect. Urinary hesitation and retention are especially distressing for males. Reducing the dose or changing to a different antipsychotic medication is the usual course of action. Constipation is a problem, especially for the elderly client. There may be a time during the acute psychotic phase of illness that a client is not tuned into his own physical discomfort, and an impaction may result. Monitoring toileting, as well as providing increased water, juices, fruits, and bran, is often helpful. Do remember to increase fluids when adding bran so that the client does not become constipated. Sometimes mild laxatives are needed temporarily. It is helpful to remember that the anticholinergic drying effect is experienced throughout the body. For example, clients with contact lenses may need additional artificial tears to relieve the discomfort they experience. Some clients may not be able to wear the contacts for awhile. Dry skin plus institutional soaps can promote skin irritation. Nasal congestion is often ignored, or the client takes cold remedies that often have an additional drying effect. Inhibited ejaculation is both an anticholinergic and an endocrine problem. This can cause problems in the client's personal life, especially if he does not relate it to the medication. A change to a different antipsychotic medication usually relieves the problem. Anhidrosis, the inability to perspire, causes an uncommon drying effect. Since perspiring is a natural cooling mechanism for the body, the client, if very warm and unable to perspire, is a candidate for heatstroke. Red, hot, dry skin and the client's complaint of discomfort are warnings for the health provider to immediately remove him to a cooler area. The same kind of first aid procedures used for pending heat stroke are in order.

Another important group of side effects are the *allergic* side effects, which include urticaria (rash), photosensitivity, contact dermatitis, and, less commonly, jaundice, agranulocytosis, and hyperpigmentation. If the rash is mild, a dermatological lotion may be enough to give relief. Otherwise, lowering the dosage or changing to a different antipsychotic medication is necessary. Clients with photosensitivity burn quickly in the sun. Sun screens with a factor of about 15 are helpful, as are long sleeves and a large-brimmed hat. Sometimes the client must stay indoors until his body adjusts to the medication. Contact dermatitis is caused by direct contact with a liquid antipsychotic medication. A rash at the corners of the mouth may indicate involvement of the mucous membranes in the mouth. Adequate dilution of the medication is necessary, and taking the medication through a straw is another safeguard. The health provider who dispenses the medication is also susceptible, the most common contact being with spilled medication on the outside of the bottle. Historically, this has always been the fault of the previous shift for not wiping off the bottle! Some health providers become so sensitive that they must wear rubber gloves to dispense liquid medication. Fortunately, drug-induced jaundice and agranulocytosis are rare. Drug-induced jaundice often begins with a flu-like syndrome (Kline and Davis, 1973:58). Agranulocytosis also seems to be an allergic response that occurs during the first two months of treatment. "Sore throat and high fever are early symptoms of agranulocytosis" (Kline and Davis:58). Hyperpigmentation is another rare, but interesting, side effect in which the skin develops a blue-gray or purple discoloration.

This occurs only after long-term treatment with high doses of chlorpromazine (Kline and Davis:58). Discontinuing the medication usually reverses the symptoms of any of the allergic side effects.

Other side effects do occur. For example, ocular changes, such as blurred vision and difficulty with accommodation (focusing), make it more difficult for the client to read or participate in games. Usually the problem is mild, and instructing the client to focus longer on what he is looking at seems to help. Mellaril, however, in high doses can occasionally cause pigmentary retinopathy, which can lead to blindness. Although such cases are rare, the health provider must be alert to clients' complaints that things look brownish to him (Mason and Granacher, 1980:238). Chlorpromazine (Thorazine) can cause opacity of the lens and cornea, but it does not lead to blindness (Kline and Davis, 1973:58). Endocrine side effects, depending on the client's presenting problem, can add to his anxiety. Some of the symptoms mimic pregnancy: breast enlargement, lactation, lack of menses, weight gain, and a false-positive pregnancy test. Men can also experience inhibited ejaculation and altered libido. Water intoxication may result from a client's attempts to relieve a dry mouth or by inappropriate secretion of the antidiuretic hormone. Changing to a different antipsychotic agent is often effective. Although the medications share side effects, one medication will exhibit a higher level of some side effects than another. Paradoxical effects can also occur, and the client responds with increased symptoms. Initially, this may be difficult to identify. And, since the client looks more psychotic, he is often given an additional dose of medication, which, of course, increases the symptoms.

As a class, antipsychotic medications are safe and highly effective. Yet approximately 60 percent of clients discontinue their medications. One reason seems to be that although the client is free of psychotic symptoms, he continues to experience some residual side effects. Because the antipsychotic agents are long-acting, the antipsychotic effect remains, and the side effects disappear first. By the time symptoms of the illness reappear, the client does not connect them with discontinuing medication. "Ayd (1966), [who] coined the term 'drug holiday' for intermittent drug free schedules, initiated a 'never-on-Sunday' policy for his chronically ill patients on maintenance antipsychotic therapy" (Mason and Granacher, 1980:84). It proved to be safe and effective. He added days off and varied them. This is one of the partial solutions being used by health providers who work with chronically ill clients. The result often is that of greater compliance. The client has some sense of control of his own life. He feels he is improving and is not entirely dependent on medication.

Antipsychotic Agents

Trade Name	Generic Name
Compazine	prochlorperazine
Haldol	haloperidol
Loxitane	loxaprine
Mellaril	thioridazine
Moban	molindone
Navane	thiothixene
Prolixin	fluphenazine
Prolixin Decanoate or Enanthate (long acting intramuscular injection)	fluphenazine decanoate or enanthate
Quide	piperacetazine
Serentil	mesoridazine
Stelazine	trifluoperazine
Taractan	chlorprothixene
Thorazine	chlorpromazine
Trilafon	perphenazine
Vesprin	triflupromazine

Anticholinergic Agents

Trade Name	Generic Name
Akineton	biperiden HCl
Artane	trihexyphenidyl HCl
Benadryl	diphenhydramine HCl
Cogentin	benztropine mesylate
Kemadrin	procyclidine HCl

ANTIANXIETY AGENTS

Antianxiety agents, previously known as minor tranquilizers, primarily relieve anxiety and muscle tension. They differ from the antipsychotic agents in significant ways. For example, they lack antipsychotic activity, no matter how large the dose. They also lack antiemetic activity and do not have significant anticholinergic effects or extrapyramidal symptoms. Consequently, clients tend to prefer these agents because they relieve the uncomfortable anxiety and muscular tension, usually without producing significant side effects. Ideally, these medications are used to relieve high levels of anxiety and tension and yet leave the client with sufficient anxiety to motivate him to seek a solution to the actual problem.

These medications also have an anticonvulsive action, and they are useful during alcohol detoxification in preventing or decreasing the intensity of end-stage withdrawal symptoms. Since these medications are CNS depressants, they produce an additive effect when combined with other CNS depressants. For example, combining an antianxiety agent with alcohol, barbiturates, narcotics, or other drugs that depress the CNS can result in a combined effect that is greater than the sum of the two effects. The combination will affect the client as though he had ingested a larger amount of the CNS depressants. It is, in fact, a way that some individuals overdose accidentally. The most common side effects are often limited to drowsiness, fatigue, and ataxia. Confusion, however, is a significant side effect among the elderly. Occasionally, paradoxical behavioral changes are experienced, and the individual becomes agitated, hostile, or irritable. Sleep patterns can be disturbed by the onset of nightmares. Depression is a rare side effect, as are blood dyscrasias, jaundice, skin rash, hypotension, slurred speech, and blurry vision. The most common problem associated with chronic use of anxiety agents is drug dependence. This is an insidious side effect often caused by using the agent past the point for which it is prescribed, or by increasing dosages on one's own (i.e., in an attempt to use the medication as a solution to felt difficulties). Clients develop a psychic or a physical drug dependence, the psychic dependence being most common. Clients with a psychic dependence feel they need to have the medication to function, but do not experience physical effects from its withdrawal. "Withdrawal symptoms are more likely after high doses, but can also occur after usual therapeutic doses, so gradual tapering is recommended. With long-acting drugs, such as diazepam (Valium), withdrawal symptoms may be delayed for days and then be confused with anxiety" (Medical Letter, 1983:46). Withdrawal symptoms include insomnia, diaphoresis, nausea, irritability, twitching, and convulsions.

The antianxiety agents are effective and useful medications when used properly. They are meant to be used temporarily as the client pursues his treatment goals and attempts to find more effective ways to deal with stress-producing problems.

Antianxiety Agents

TRADE NAME	GENERIC NAME
Atarax	hydroxyzine
Ativan	lorazepam
Centrax	prazepam
Librium	chlordiazepoxide
Paxipam	halazepam
Serax	oxazepam
Tranxene	chlordiazepate
Valium	diazepam
Xanax	alprazolam

ANTIDEPRESSIVE AGENTS

Depression is the most common mental disorder, and it is thought that at least 10 per cent of the population will experience a major depression in their lifetime. Only about one half of those experiencing a major depression are treated and about 10 per cent of those diagnosed as having major depression commit suicide.

The tricyclic antidepressants and newer agents with different chemical structure but similar action and effectiveness are the first line of treatment for depression. As a class, these agents are considered safe and effective when used as directed. The key to success is to treat clients with sufficient medication for a long enough period of time. The health provider must be familiar with idiosyncrasies specific to this classification, in order to support the client in taking his medication. The antidepressive agents take from one to four weeks for onset of the antidepressive effect. Side effects tend to show up rapidly, and although the body builds a tolerance to most side effects in a week or two, the client may initially experience depression plus side effects. The client may fear that he is being treated improperly. Excellent instruction and support by the provider are essential to prevent the client from discontinuing his medication. Major side effects resulting from these medications fall into three general categories: (1) *anticholinergic effects* (dry mouth, constipation, dilation of the pupils, urinary hesitancy or retention, loss of accommodation of the lens of the eye, tachycardia, and, in high doses, delirium); (2) *orthostatic hypotension,* which can result in serious falls, especially among the elderly; and (3) *sedation* (drowsiness or sleepiness). Infrequent side effects include activation of a manic type of process, visual hallucinations and delusions, blood dyscrasias, allergic dermatitis, photosensitivity, gastrointestinal symptoms, and muscle tremors. Ways of dealing with potentially annoying side effects are included in the narrative on antipsychotic agents.

The antidepressive agents, with the exception of protriptyline (Vivactil), are often ordered as a single dose at bedtime (Greist and Jefferson, 1984:45). In this way, side effects occur while the client is asleep. For example, a sedating side effect may help to promote sleep. The dosage is individualized according to the client's needs and reaction to the medication. Overdose with these medications can be lethal.

The health provider needs to work closely with the client from the onset of medication therapy to explain the action of the medication, the expected time of onset, the body's adjustment to side effects, and effective management of the side effects that remain. An ever-present danger in early antidepressant therapy is suicide. The client receiving medication is able to channel his energy to formulate and implement a suicide plan before his depression significantly improves.

Another group of antidepressants are the monoamine oxidase inhibitor (MAOI) antidepressants. MAOIs inhibit the oxidase enzyme that breaks down monoamine transmitters at many places in the body, including the intestine. This results in a greater availability of these transmitters for improved message transmission in the brain. Clients who are receiving MAOIs need to be cautioned about ingesting products that would cause a significant additional supply of monoamines. Some foods contain significant amounts of tyramine, a monoamine that affects blood pressure. Large amounts of tyramine can lead to a hypertensive crisis (an extreme elevation in blood pressure), leading to rupture of blood vessels that results in a cerebrovascular accident (stroke). The client needs instruction on foods to avoid, which include the following:

avocado	meat extract
banana	pickles
caffeine (coffee, chocolate, some soft drinks)	raisins
	red wine
canned figs	salami/summer sausage
cheese (strong or aged)	smoked/aged fish, meat, or poultry
chicken livers	sour cream
concentrated yeast	soy sauce
game	yogurt
herring (kippered or pickled)	any food that causes an unusual effect

A similar reaction can occur when combining some medications with MAOIs. These medications include:

Ephedrine	Afrin
Epinephrine	Tedral
Adrenalin	Amphetamines
Isuprel	Narcotics
Neo-Synephrine	Alcohol
Norisodrine	L-Dopa
Sudafed	Aldomet

The client needs to be instructed to read labels, especially those of over-the-counter medications and combination products, and to tell his family physician that he is taking MAOIs. Other potential side effects are similar to those of the tricyclic antidepressants.

Not all clients are candidates for receiving MAOIs. Their use is reserved for symptomatic relief of depression in clients who have failed to respond satisfactorily to other antidepressant therapy. Once the MAOI antidepressant is started, the client experiences the antidepressant effect in 48 hours to three weeks. Maximum benefit is achieved within two to six weeks.

The provider's major responsibility is three-fold: (1) instruct the client about foods to avoid, (2) tell him what medications to avoid, and (3) warn him how to recognize the danger signs of an impending hypertensive crisis. "Marked elevation in blood pressure may be signaled by headache at the back of the neck, stiff neck, pounding heart beat and less frequently, nausea, vomiting and dilated pupils" (Greist and Jefferson:54). Monitoring of blood pressure on a regular basis at the onset of medication is usual in the institutional setting.

Antidepressive Agents

TRADE NAME	GENERIC NAME
Asendin	amoxapine
Aventyl	nortriptyline
Desyrel	trazodone
Elavil	amitriptyline
Ludiomil	maprotiline
Norpramin, Pertofrane	desipramine
Sinequan	doxepin
Surmontil	trimipramine maleate
Tofranil	imipramine
Vivactil	protriptyline

MAOI Antidepressant Agents

TRADE NAME	GENERIC NAME
Marplan	isocarboxazid
Nardil	phenelzine
Parnate	tranylcypromine

ANTIMANIC AGENTS

The antimanic classification is made up of one medication, lithium carbonate. "Lithium is the drug of choice for patients with mania and for long term maintenance to prevent both depressive and manic episodes in bipolar disorder" (Medical Letter, 1983:48). Lithium was first determined to be effective in the treatment of manic disorder in the late 1940s. However, it was not approved for use in the United States until the 1970s because of lithium intoxication–related deaths during the time that lithium chloride salt was being used as a salt substitute.

Although toxicity is severe, lithium can be administered safely if the serum lithium level is monitored (Medical Letter, 1983:48). To get an accurate reading, the blood sample must be drawn 12 hours after the last dose of lithium. The best time for this is in the morning, and the morning dose must be held until blood is drawn. Once lithium therapy is started, the serum level is usually monitored three times a week until the client has stabilized. A serum level of 1.2–1.6 milliequivalents per liter (mEq/L) is considered therapeutic for most clients, although individual sensitivity to lithium varies. The risk of toxicity increases above 2 mEq/L. Once the client's condition is stabilized, medication is reduced to bring the serum level to 0.8 to 1.2 mEq/L for maintenance. Weekly and then monthly serum levels are required indefinitely (Mason and Granacher, 1980:261).

It takes approximately two to three weeks for a therapeutic effect with lithium therapy. Consequently, the client will usually receive temporary treatment with an antipsychotic medication until the therapeutic blood level of lithium is obtained. Nausea and fatigue are common side effects that can occur early in the therapy. Tremor, thirst, edema, and weight gain may be present throughout the therapy. Confusion is an important toxic side effect that may be missed (Medical Letter, 1983:48). Other toxic symptoms include ataxia, impaired coordination, dizziness, headache, blurred vision, muscle weakness, and gastrointestinal symptoms. Untreated, lithium intoxication can lead to coma and death. Impaired renal function, decreased sodium intake, and diuretic therapy provide a risk for toxicity. In order to prevent toxicity, it is important to understand the relationship between lithium and sodium. Lithium and sodium share similar chemical characteristics. The sites for absorption of both are in the kidney, where some of each drug is absorbed and some is excreted. As long as the sodium intake and output remain the same, the lithium absorption and excretion will be stable. However, anything that changes this balance will have an inverse effect on the lithium. For example, a low-salt diet or diuretics will result in more lithium absorption sites in the kidney. This can result in toxicity, since more lithium is now being absorbed. More salt in the diet can result in fewer lithium absorption sites, and this can result in the return of manic symptoms. This points out the need for the client to know as much about his medication as possible so that he will see the physician for medication adjustment any time he experiences major changes in his life style. Even though treatment with lithium is 80 per cent effective, approximately 60 per cent of clients discontinue the medication on their own. Clients frequently complain of "feeling low." Clearly, there is a need for additional therapy to help the client learn to adjust to his new affect. The client also needs to learn all about his medication and the role it plays in his life, since lithium is generally prescribed as a lifetime treatment.

Antimanic Agents

Trade Name	Generic Name
Eskalith, Lithane, Lithonate	lithium carbonate

OTHER PHYSICAL/MEDICAL THERAPIES

Some physical/medical or somatic therapies that were used prior to the introduction of psychiatric medications for treating psychiatric problems included electroconvulsive therapy, insulin coma therapy, psychosurgery, and physiotherapy.

ELECTROCONVULSIVE THERAPY

Electroconvulsive therapy (ECT), also known as electroshock therapy (EST), was described by Cerletti and Bini in 1938 as a method of treating certain types of psychiatric disorders. It is most effective with clients who are severely depressed and/or compulsively suicidal.

The administration of ECT has been greatly improved to the point that sometimes the only way one can tell that a client is having a seizure is by monitoring his brain waves with an electroencephalogram (EEG). The treatment consists of the passage of a small, carefully controlled electric current between two electrodes applied to the head. In bilateral treatment, one electrode is applied to each side of the head; in unilateral treatment, both electrodes are applied to the same side of the head, usually the right side or the less dominant side. With unilateral treatment, less confusion and memory loss seem to occur, although usually both of these effects are temporary.

The treatment is given in a specially equipped room. Prior to treatment, the client receives an injection to reduce secretions in the mouth. Treatments are usually given before breakfast. Clothing must be loose; jewelry, eye glasses, dentures, and other prosthetic devices should be removed. The client should be reminded to void before the treatment. Once in the treatment room, the client is given an anesthetic, and sleep occurs very quickly. He is then given an intravenous medication to produce muscular relaxation. The client should have no awareness of any discomfort; he does not feel the electric current and usually has no memory of the treatment. The treatment produces generalized muscular contractions of a convulsive nature. Sometimes these contractions, which last only about 60 seconds, are barely visible. Shortly after, the client slowly awakens and may experience some confusion similar to someone coming out of any type of brief anesthesia. When the client is ready, he can be up and about, eat, and return to his room. The number and frequency of treatments vary with the condition being treated, the individual response to treatment, and the psychiatrist giving the treatments. An average course of therapy may include four to ten treatments (Task Force Report 14, APA, 1978:174–175).

Electroconvulsive therapy is considered a surgical procedure and therefore requires a complete physical examination and informed consent from the client and/or his guardian. "Indeed, for a procedure that has a very good record of safety, regulations of ECT are far more extensive than are those applied to brain surgery, open heart surgery, and many other bodily invasions that are far more dangerous" (Greenblatt, 1984:1409). What actually occurs as a result of electroconvulsive therapy remains unknown; however, it is quite certain that changes occur in the neurochemistry of the brain.

Electroconvulsive therapy remains one of the most effective means of treating severe clinical depression. A positive, supportive attitude on the part of the health provider is important in allaying the anxiety that clients may experience while receiving somatic therapies.

Insulin Coma Therapy

Insulin coma therapy, sometimes referred to as insulin shock treatment, was introduced by Manfred Sakel in 1933 for the treatment of schizophrenia. The amount of insulin in the blood stream determines the rate of oxidation of carbohydrates; therefore, the injection of a large amount of insulin into the body will greatly reduce the sugar content of the blood, producing hypoglycemia. As the brain cells are deprived of glucose, their principal fuel, a loss of consciousness and coma occur. The treatment is begun with small doses of insulin, 10 to 15 units, which are increased daily until the desired depth of coma is attained.

With the advent of psychiatric medication, use of the cumbersome insulin coma therapy, which required very skilled practitioners, declined rapidly.

Psychosurgery

A surgical procedure consisting of a severance of the connection between the thalamus and frontal lobe is known as a prefrontal lobotomy. It was developed in 1935 by Egas Moniz, a Portuguese neurologist who received the Nobel Prize in Medicine in 1949 for his work in prefrontal lobotomy (Kolb and Brodie, 1982:844). The prefrontal lobotomy is considered a radical procedure that was undertaken only after other forms of treatment were unsuccessful. One of this writer's observations was that a lobotomy's success was related, in part, to postoperative care. It was important to engage the client in a "total push" rehabilitation program that involved a re-education program, including the activities of daily living.

A variation of the prefrontal lobotomy, the transorbital lobotomy, was introduced into the United States by Drs. Walter Freeman and James Watt. The "ice-pick–like" instrument (Kalinowsky and Hoch, 1961:281) used for the procedure made it possible to perform the surgery in the doctor's office; however, the intensive rehabilitation program that was present with inpatient care did not occur on an outpatient basis. The transorbital procedure has been abandoned, and the few lobotomies that are still performed are carried out through open craniotomies by neurosurgeons (Kolb and Brodie, 1982: 844). One of the results of the lobotomy was a decrease in the intensity of the individual's affect. When tranquilizers were first introduced, they were sometimes referred to as "chemical lobotomies," since a calming of the affect occurred. The calming, however, was not permanent, as in the lobotomy.

PHYSIOTHERAPY

One of the most common methods of treating persons who were mentally ill prior to the introduction of psychiatric medications was hydrotherapy. This form of treatment consisted of a continuing hot water bath or of cold wet sheet packs. Both treatments were very soothing to the excited and agitated client. In the cold wet sheet pack, the client was wrapped mummy-fashion in two wet sheets that were thoroughly wrung out. Care was taken that no two skin surfaces touched and that no pockets of air were left in the wrapping. When the entire body was suddenly cooled, the immediate action was for the cutaneous blood vessels to contract, resulting in a feeling of comfortable warmth, relaxation, and drowsiness. The client's physical condition, pulse, color, and general reaction, needed to be checked at regular intervals.

REFERENCES

APA, 1978. Task Force Report 14: Electroconvulsive Therapy. Washington, D.C., American Psychiatric Association.

Cochran, C.C., 1984. A change of mind about ECT. Am J Nurs, Vol. 84, No. 8, pp. 1004–1005.

Dienhart, P., 1983. Drug therapy alters the practice of psychiatry. Health Service, University of Minnesota, Minneapolis, Spring, pp. 10–14.

Fink, M., 1984. Meduna and the origins of convulsive therapy. Am J Psychiatry, Vol. 141, No. 9, September, pp. 1034–1041.

Gilman, A., Goodman, L., and Gilman, A., 1980. Goodman and Gilman's The Pharmacological Basis of Therapeutics. 6th ed. New York, Macmillan Publishers.

Greenblatt, M., 1984. ECT: Please, no more regulations! Am J Psychiatry, Vol. 141 No. 11, pp. 1409–1410.

Greist, J., and Jefferson, J., 1984. Depression and Its Treatment: Help for the Nation's #1 Mental Problem. Washington, D.C., American Psychiatric Association Press.

Kalinowsky, L.B., and Hock, P.A., 1961. Somatic Treatments in Psychiatry. New York, Grune and Stratton.

Kolb, L., and Brodie, K., 1982. Modern Clinical Psychiatry. 3rd ed. Philadelphia, W.B. Saunders Co.

Kline, N., and Davis, J., 1973. Psychotropic drugs. Am J Nurs, Vol. 73, No. 1, pp. 54–62.

Mason, A., and Granacher, R., 1980. Clinical Handbook of Antipsychotic Drug Therapy. New York, Brunner/Mazel.

Medical Letter, 1983. Drugs for psychiatric disorders. May 13, Vol. 25, No. 635, pp. 45–51.

O'Connell, R., 1982. A review of the use of electroconvulsive therapy. Am J Psychiatry, Vol. 33, No. 6, pp. 469–473.

Ratcliff, J.D., 1983. I Am Joe's Body, New York, Berkley Books.

Thomas, S., 1978. The uses and abuses of electroconvulsive shock therapy. J Psychosoc Nurs Ment Health Serv, November, pp. 17–23.

Weiner, R., 1984. Convulsive therapy: 50 years later. Am J Psychiatry. Vol. 141, No. 9, p. 1079.

Wilson, H., and Kneisl, C., 1979. Psychiatric Nursing, Menlo Park, CA. Addison-Wesley Publishers, Inc.

APPLIED BEHAVIOR ANALYSIS (BEHAVIOR MANAGEMENT)*

LEARNING OBJECTIVES—Upon completing this chapter, the reader will be able to:

1. Define four principles of behavior.

2. List an application for each behavior principle.

This chapter is designed to introduce the health provider to the discipline of applied behavior analysis. This discipline is often referred to as the field of behavior management, a "down-to-earth approach" to behavior change. The behavior principles introduced in this section can be systematically applied to reinstate, increase, maintain, teach, or decrease the behavior of individuals in short- or long-term health care facilities.

The pictures in Figure 14–1 portray a small segment of life. By answering the questions below, the health provider can find out what has happened to each person.

1. What did the health providers do when Bill interrupted their conversation?
2. What happened to Bill when he interrupted the health providers?
3. What happened to the health providers after they responded to Bill's interruption?

The provider has just been exposed to behavior analysis. Increasingly, more individuals and facilities are turning to applied behavior analysis because it utilizes techniques that account for behavior in an objective format.

WHAT IS APPLIED BEHAVIOR ANALYSIS?

Applied behavior analysis is the systematic application of the principles of behavior (Sulzer-Azaroff/Mayer, 1977).

In applied behavior analysis:
1. Behavior change focuses on the here and now. Developmental history, intelligence, and other factors are considered important; however, primary emphasis is on what the individual is doing in his current environment.
2. There is a search for lawful relationships in behavior. An emphasis is on

---

*This chapter was written by Paula Lamberg, Behavior Analyst.

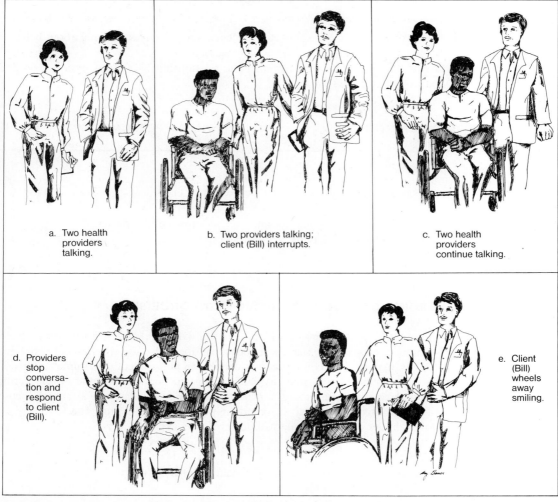

a. Two health providers talking.

b. Two providers talking; client (Bill) interrupts.

c. Two health providers continue talking.

d. Providers stop conversation and respond to client (Bill).

e. Client (Bill) wheels away smiling.

Figure 14-1. An interaction between health providers and a client.

identifying what factors are currently maintaining the problem behavior. Applied behavior analysis as a science is a study of "what is":

—What behaviors are you attempting to change?

—What measurements are you going to use?

—What consequences can be changed?

—What variable might be changed to see what the effect would be?

3. The focus is on changing the problem behavior. Behaviors are defined in terms that are observable, measurable, and precise. This is emphasized by the primary authors in Unit II, Chapter 5.

4. There is a focus on the individual, not on groups of people. Behavior analysis programs are custom fit to the unique problems of the individual. Specificity is the rule of thumb.

5. There is an ongoing process in which behavioral objectives are progressively reanalyzed as time goes on.

6. Methods can be designed so that clients have input into the decision-making process and informed consent is obtained before initiating the program. Where needed, guardians or relatives can approve the approaches and goals.

A formula for applied behavior analysis is:

Behavior Procedure + Measurement + Evaluation = Applied Behavior Analysis

A behavior procedure is the application of behavior principles to bring about behavior change.

A behavior principle is a rule describing the relationship between what a person does and a specific condition.

SPECIFIC CONDITION	WHAT A PERSON DOES
Hears a funny joke ------------------------>	Laughs
Feels something in his throat ---------------->	Coughs
Eats a big meal ------------------------>	Secretes gastric juices
Receives a pay raise --------------------->	Jumps up and down

Laughing, coughing, secreting gastric juices, and jumping up and down all follow a certain behavior or event. What follows a behavior is called a consequence.

INCREASING BEHAVIOR: POSITIVE REINFORCEMENT

A strong case could be presented for the position that the single most important factor causing human behavior is the consequence of the behavior. Because of individual backgrounds, many people connect consequence with punishment. It is important to note that other consequences are readily available. Consequences can be good or reinforcing, bad or punishing, or neutral (things remaining the same). A behavioral approach focuses primarily on consequences that are good or positively reinforcing. The following are everyday examples of what people will do for consequences:

1. Work for money.
2. Take shelter for protection from cold weather.
3. Study for good grades.
4. Wait for a speeding car to pass to avoid being hit.
5. Save for retirement.
6. Swim to prevent drowning.

We learn from the effects of our behavior.

If a client repeatedly experiences some pleasant effect immediately following a particular behavior, he tends to repeat that behavior. A client who is reinforced with verbal praise is more likely to assist the health provider with an activity if following the activity the health provider comments, "Thanks so much, I really appreciate your help." The next time the provider begins the same activity, it is likely that the client will return to assist. This is known as the principle of positive reinforcement.

Definition of Positive Reinforcement:
When a stimulus (object or event) follows a behavior, the strength or rate of that behavior increases or remains constant.

The only way to tell whether a consequence is reinforcing is to observe its effect on the behavior it follows. This is a very critical point because consequences that are reinforcing for one individual may not be effective, positive reinforcers for another. Some people would walk a mile for a piece of candy; others would not take the candy if it were given to them free of charge. There is a difference between this definition of *positive reinforcement* and the general use of the term *reward*. You do not proclaim something to be a reinforcer;

it is determined by the rate of responding or its effect on the behavior it follows. For example, Mary has just completed making her bed, a task she rarely completes unassisted. The health provider gives her a graham cracker as a reinforcer. The next day Mary does not make her bed. The provider then states to Mary, "If you help me make your bed, you can have a graham cracker." Still, Mary only observes. Is the graham cracker a reward, proclaimed by the health provider, or a reinforcer? In this case, the cracker is a reward because it does not maintain or increase the frequency of bed-making. No matter what the provider's intentions, a consequence is a positive reinforcer only if it maintains or increases the behavior it follows. The name of the game is finding out what things the individual will respond to.

What can be done to discover possible reinforcers for an individual?

1. Ask the client what he enjoys doing.
2. Observe what the client does in his leisure time.
3. Observe what available activities or outings a client attends.
4. Observe with whom the client talks.
5. Offer a pair of reinforcers and observe which one the client selects.
6. Ask the client to fill out a reinforcer survey (a list of events, activities, edibles, etc.).

The following is a small sample list of possible no-cost or low-cost positive reinforcers:

Social	Activity	Material/Edible
kind word	housekeeping tasks	magazines
hug	mending	letters
friendly smile	collating papers	clothes
nod	running errands	hobby supplies
wink	setting tables	work displayed
pat on back	assisting with groups	certificates
hand shake	serving nourishments	ribbons
coffee with a supervisor	movement games	stickers
phone call	reading	cosmetics
	hobbies	beverages
	window shopping	gum/candy/cookies
	free community events	cigarettes

A case could be made not only for the position that consequences are the single most important factor causing behavior, but that social reinforcers, such as the kind listed above, are very important consequences that maintain behavior.

Your contact with a person has an important effect on his behavior.

Often, the only time a person is noticed is when he is either doing something wrong or not doing anything at all. For example:

—"Come on, eat just a spoonful. Let's eat all our food if we want to stay good and healthy."
—"Let's go now. Come on, let's not be late; let's go."
—"I've told you the last six times I responded to your call bell, don't ring the bell for every little thing. I told you I make rounds every half hour; that's when I can answer any questions."
—"Now comb your hair. Everyday I have to remind you to comb your hair; don't you want to look pretty?"

Health providers are often puzzled with recurring problem behaviors such as those mentioned above. What can be done to change problem behaviors? First, the target behavior—the behavior to be changed—must be identified. This is done in precise, observable, and measurable terms. Then, the consequences that follow the target behavior must be identified. The previous examples could be illustrated as follows:

PROBLEM BEHAVIOR	**CONSEQUENCE**
Eating small amounts of food during meals ------>	Coaxing/assisting
Going to an activity late ------------------>	Coaxing
Frequent use of call bell ------------------>	Answering call bell
Uncombed hair ---------------------------->	Coaxing

The coaxing, assisting, and answering are forms of attention or social reinforcement. Attention can be a very powerful reinforcer; therefore, the attention may be what is maintaining the very behavior you are attempting to eliminate. Positive reinforcement can maintain both desirable and undesirable behavior.

It is now time to change strategies! If attention is a reinforcer, observing a client performing a desirable behavior should be a cue to respond (e.g., "Thanks" or "That's great"). Now attention is focused on praising accomplishment and reinforcing achievement.

Mark Twain put it this way: "I can live two months on a good compliment."

A quick compliment, a timely nod, or an appreciative word are small investments that may have large payoffs.

A special form of positive reinforcement is the Premack Principle, often referred to as "Grandma's Rule." Grandma used to say, "Eat your vegetables before you can have your dessert." What grandma was saying is that first you must do what you don't really want to do before you do something you like to do.

Behaviors that a client does quite often can be used as reinforcement for behaviors that seldom occur. The Premack Principle utilizes only activities as reinforcers, thus providing health providers with a practical and convenient tool for behavior change.

Some other possible examples of the Premack Principle, or Grandma's Rule, are:

1. Take your meds, then receive some recreation time.
2. Wash up, then go to the game room.
3. Clean off the work table before leaving.
4. Complete your assignment before break.
5. After five minutes of leg exercises, you can make your phone call.

The following are key points in using positive reinforcement most effectively.

1. Immediacy. Positive reinforcement must immediately follow the desired behavior. The faster a reinforcer is given after the behavior, the more effective it will be. The client learns what behavior is being reinforced. The health provider who comments how well the client eats during mealtime (while he is actually eating) will reinforce the client more effectively than the health provider who waits until afternoon rounds to compliment the client on how well he ate.

2. Consistency. Positive reinforcement must be delivered consistently by all health providers across all shifts. The client learns which of his behaviors lead to reinforcement and which do not. Behaviors to be reinforced and the reinforcement procedure should be clearly specified in the patient's total plan of care.

3. Specific Praise. In certain cases, the delivery of positive reinforcement, especially in the form of praise, should be paired with the specific reason for its delivery. For example, rather than saying, "You did a good job," you could say, "You did a good job filing the charts in the correct folders." Specific praise is focused on that aspect of the behavior that deserves it. Emphasis is on the behavior, not the person, which is important. Then, when praise is withheld for an undesirable behavior, the client learns that it is his behavior that is unacceptable, not him as an individual.

4. Deprivation. It is important to take into account the deprivation level of the reinforcer to be used. A client who is not thirsty is unlikely to do anything to obtain a drink. Crackers that are available three times a day at nourishment time may not be effective reinforcers at other times. Deprivation, or how long it has been since the reinforcer was last delivered, plays an important role in ensuring reinforcer effectiveness.

5. Novelty. People find experiencing novel or new objects or events reinforcing. Christmas and birthdays with wrapped packages testify to this! Some examples of novel reinforcers are a "surprise box" containing objects or slips of paper listing different activities; and a "job jar," which varies the order of daily tasks. Satiation, or "getting filled" on large amounts of one reinforcer, is not a concern when varying reinforcers and using novel reinforcers.

6. Sampling. "Try it; you'll like it." Sometimes a person is unfamiliar with an object or has not experienced an event; therefore, its potential reinforcing properties are unknown. Grocery stores give out free samples with the hope that customers will like the product and will purchase it. Sampling also helps discover possible reinforcers. Displaying a new magazine, starting a new activity, or teaching part of a new game are examples of reinforcer sampling. Once the person begins to enjoy an experience, it becomes a reinforcer for him.

7. Contingencies. After identifying powerful, positive reinforcers, those same reinforcers can be utilized to bring about behavior change. "If you complete your exercise program, you can go to the lounge." "If you attend three in-house activities this week, you can go for a van ride on the weekend." These are "if . . . then" contingencies. If a person does a particular behavior, then he will receive reinforcement. If he does not do the behavior, he will not receive the reinforcement. Reinforcement is contingent upon performance of a specific behavior.

8. Scheduling. If a health provider is trying to teach a client a new routine, the more often the client's behavior is reinforced, the better. The health provider may decide to teach a client to pick up after himself. As part of the approach, the provider may ask him to put his dirty clothes in a hamper. Each time he does so, the provider may praise him. When teaching a new behavior or reinstating a behavior, it is important to reinforce the behavior each time it occurs. This is called *continuous reinforcement*. After a behavior is fairly well-established by continuous reinforcement, the frequency of reinforcement can be reduced. Reinforcing some, but not all responses, is called an intermittent schedule of reinforcement. *Intermittent reinforcement* is most effective in maintaining behavior. Once the new routine is learned, and dirty clothes are always being placed in the hamper, praise for performing this behavior can then be delivered occasionally.

9. Tokens. There are times when it is simply not possible to immediately deliver a reinforcer. Using some tangible item can solve this problem and help bridge the delay between the behavior and the reinforcer. Money can "bridge the gap." It can be earned for a certain behavior, saved, then exchanged for a desired object or activity at a later time. In clinical settings, tokens can function as money. Tokens can be points, checks, slips of paper, chips, or other tangible items that can be accumulated and traded in. Token reinforcement systems are often used with individuals who do not respond to praise or attention. It is useful to pair praise with delivery of the token so eventually the provider can phase out the token and the behavior will be maintained with praise or social reinforcement alone. In health care facilities, tokens can be exchanged for a pass, a community activity, edibles, extra visits with the health provider, or whatever has an impact on the client's behavior.

Many of the problems that confront health providers in changing clients' behaviors can be handled by means of *contingent positive reinforcement*. The search for effective reinforcers may require some creativity and flexibility; however, effective reinforcers can be found for everyone. It is important to note that if a behavior ceases, it is not the fault of the client or the health provider. Rather, it is then time to re-analyze the conditions (e.g., immediacy, consistency, schedules, etc.) that are known to influence reinforcer effectiveness.

One major advantage of a behavioral approach is that it can be applied easily and rapidly, leading to behavior change. With the background from this section on positive reinforcement, a person is ready to start applying these behavior principles to bring about behavior change. The principles presented in the remainder of this section add sophistication to the techniques to change behavior.

Increasing Behavior: Shaping—A Positive Approach

> First things first.
> Great oaks from little acorns grow.
> One must walk before he runs.
> You can build big things, a brick at a time.

As a ceramic pot must be shaped from a lump of clay, so a new behavior must be shaped from an existing behavior.

Definition of Shaping:
Shaping is the procedure used to teach a complex behavior using small steps. This is done by reinforcing responses that approximate more and more the final, sought-after behavior.

When a person fails to reach his goal, how many times has he given up? The reasons for these failures can, to a great extent, be attributed to attempting too large a task.

The following are key points in using shaping effectively:

1. Start at the client's current level of behavior. The health provider must work with the client at the client's level and shape his behavior from that point. In teaching a client to shave unassisted, it was observed that the client would pick up the razor, then stop and wait for the health provider to assist. For this client just picking up the razor was initially reinforced. Next, picking up the razor and bringing it to his face was reinforced, and so on.

2. Break the complex behavior into small steps. By breaking the complex behavior into small steps, each succeeding step gets closer to the final behavioral goal. An example of breaking a complex behavior such as washing into small steps follows:

A. Pick up soap.
B. Pick up washcloth.
C. Soap washcloth.
D. Wash face and neck.
E. Wash stomach and chest.
F. Wash arms.
G. Wash thighs and genitals.
H. Wash feet.
I. Rinse.
J. Dry.

3.   Reinforce successful completion of each step. Failure to complete a step suggests the need for smaller steps and more repetitive practice. Reinforcement reinforces all previous steps.

4.   Prompting. Rather than waiting long lengths of time for a client to begin the next step in a shaping procedure, the health provider should prompt that step. Prompts are of at least three varieties, and the use of prompts should progress from the least intrusive (verbal prompt) to modeling prompt, and, if required, to the physical guidance prompts. The following are examples of these three prompts:

Verbal prompt: "Pick up your spoon."

Modeling or demonstrative prompt: "Watch as I pick up my spoon, then pick up yours in exactly the same way."

Physical guidance prompt: The health provider places his hand on top of the client's hand, and together they pick up the spoon. (A physical guidance prompt is often combined with a verbal prompt.)

Once the behavior is learned, it is important to gradually phase out or remove the prompts so constant reminders and suggestions are no longer required.

5.   Reaching the goal is not enough. It is crucial to take the newly acquired behavior and strengthen it with positive reinforcement. Once firmly established, an approach can then be developed to maintain the behavior.

Shaping is a procedure that can aid health providers in teaching clients new behaviors that will promote independent functioning.

Reducing Behavior: Extinction—A Positive Approach

There may be many undesirable or peculiar behaviors that the health provider observes every day in the work setting, such as recurring physical complaints, temper tantrums, excessive office visits, nagging/begging, persistent questioning, peculiar talk, unusual gestures, and junk collecting. The health provider may be perplexed by such behaviors, behaviors often thought of as unaccountable. Are these behaviors unaccountable, or could they possibly be maintained by some form of consequence?

Situations arise in which a person would like to give a little extra attention or a small gift to make up for or get rid of an unpleasant behavior (e.g., pick up a child to silence a temper tantrum, dismiss a rowdy group, give a quarter to a person who lost his money). However, the attention of picking up the child may actually be a positive reinforcer for the tantrum behavior and may increase the probability of additional temper tantrums. Likewise, dismissing a rowdy group may be a strong reinforcer for some members of the group. In the same way, replacing the lost quarter could actually be reinforcing "careless" behavior. Consider another situation in which two people are arguing, and one runs and tells. The consequence is lots of attention. Throughout this section it has been pointed out that attention can be a very powerful positive reinforcer for some individuals. However, a person may reinforce the very behavior he would like to eliminate. What can be done to change these problem behaviors?

Once the problem behavior has been identified, the consequences that follow that behavior must be identified. If attention is identified as the consequence, then attention must be discontinued for that particular behavior.

Definition of Extinction:
Extinction is the discontinuation or withdrawal of positive reinforcement for a specific behavior.

Mrs. Jones is incontinent three or four times a day. When she is discovered incontinent, the health provider talks with her as she cleans her up and changes her clothing. What has been observed is that the health provider talks with Mrs. Jones more when she is incontinent than when she is continent; therefore, the attention (conversation with the health provider) could be the reinforcing consequence maintaining the incontinence. "Ignore the bad behavior," is easier said than done. There are many techniques to use in ignoring a behavior (using an extinction procedure), and if these techniques are not used carefully, the behavior may actually get worse.

The following are key points in using extinction effectively:

1. Identify the positive reinforcers. Look at a situation from an objective, analytical standpoint (i.e., not making judgments, not questioning a person's intentions, not blaming anyone). Simply observe and record what specific consequences follow the problem behavior. Once the reinforcing consequences have been identified, a behavior program can be developed. After a thorough medical examination ruled out organic causes for Robert's persistent eye complaints, the health provider decided to use an extinction procedure. All complaints of sore eyes were ignored, although health providers were always on the alert for any possible changes in his eyes. Robert then sought out a peer who reassured him that his eyes were all right. From an objective standpoint, the attention Robert received from his peer was the reinforcer maintaining his complaining behavior.

2. Identify the specific conditions of extinction. State specifically when to ignore what behavior. For example, rather than "Ignore Robert when he complains," state, "Each time Robert complains about sore eyes, the health providers are to ignore this behavior (make no verbal comment or gesture)."

3. Communicate the procedure. Make certain all the health providers are familiar with the procedure. It is also wise to include the clients who associate with Robert so they can ignore his eye complaints as well. Never assume that someone knows what technique is being used or what changes have been made in a program.

4. Ride the crest of the wave. Eliminating a behavior takes time; therefore, maintain the extinction procedure for a sufficient length of time before evaluating the results. It takes a lot of stamina to ignore a bothersome behavior and to decide not to give in. Once you no longer allow the client to have his way, you can look for a temporary increase in the behavior before it begins to decrease. When this happens, remind yourself of the long-term payoff, and the effort will seem worthwhile.

5. Combine extinction with positive reinforcement. When ignoring one problem behavior, all other appropriate behaviors must receive abundant positive reinforcement. For example, in using an extinction procedure to decrease delusional talk, delusional talk was ignored, and all neutral, appropriate talk was reinforced with attention. Under these conditions, delusional talk dropped to a very low level, and appropriate talk increased. It must be determined before initiating an extinction procedure whether sufficient reinforcement is available to a client for his appropriate behaviors. A well-structured daily environment filled with ample opportunity to receive reinforcement goes a long way in decreasing inappropriate, attention-seeking behaviors.

Extinction can be an effective method for reducing many undesirable behaviors; however, it is a procedure to use only when behaviors will not lead to physical harm or danger. When withholding reinforcement for an undesirable behavior is not possible, an alternative reduction technique should be used.

Reducing Behavior: Reinforcing Alternative Behavior—A Positive Approach

A client frequently stands at the nursing station when health providers are busy charting. If he was attending the three o'clock activity available in the dayroom, he would not have the opportunity to stand at the nurse's station. Activity attendance is thus chosen for strengthening, and, at the same time, the client's standing at the station should decrease.

Another client spends his day isolated in his room. Assisting with setting up nourishments and running errands are behaviors that are incompatible with social isolation. Reinforcing those behaviors should decrease the amount of time the client spends alone.

A person cannot walk around with both his hands over his ears and hold a portable radio at the same time. Nor can a person lie on the floor and sit in a chair simultaneously. Reinforcing alternative behaviors and incompatible alternative behaviors are positive approaches to decrease problem behaviors. The health provider should use positive reinforcement for appropriate behavior combined with extinction for inappropriate behavior.

INTRODUCTION TO PUNISHMENT AND AVERSIVE CONTROL

Up to this point, the behavior principles introduced have been based on positive approaches to either increase or decrease behavior. The final three behavior principles, Time-Out, Response Cost, and Escape, are punitive or aversive approaches.

Since the initiation of the mental health movement, the trend has been away from punishment in the treatment of the mentally ill. However, there are two circumstances in which punishment may be required because the effects of positive reinforcement approaches would likely be slower. These circumstances are:

1. If the individual exhibits overt, self-injurious behavior, or he is a danger to others, punishment may be required.
2. If the individual's behavior is so frequent (e.g., head banging) that there is little or no incompatible behavior to reinforce, punishment may be required.

Prior to implementing procedures that involve the use of aversive stimuli, positive, alternative procedures for reducing client behavior should always be considered first. Legal, moral, and ethical issues must be considered, particularly as they relate to informed consent, institutional review, and continual program supervision. Punishment is a procedure that generally should be reserved for serious maladaptive behaviors. Positive approaches have long-lasting results, few side effects, and can be generalized to other appropriate behaviors.

Reducing Behavior: Time-Out—An Aversive Approach

Time-out is often associated with isolating a person from other people for a period of time. But isolation is not necessarily time-out, nor is time-out necessarily isolation.

Definition of Time-Out:
Time-out is any period of time, used as a consequence, during which the individual is prevented from emitting the behaviors that have been reinforced (Mertens, 1982:139).

Time-out simply refers to time out from positive reinforcement. Either the individual is removed from the reinforcing environment, or the reinforcing environment is removed from the individual for a certain length of time. These two forms of time-out are illustrated below:

BEHAVIOR	CONSEQUENCE
Yelling in dayroom ---------------------->	Removal from dayroom for 15 minutes.
Yelling in dayroom ---------------------->	Health provider leaves dayroom and client is left in a nonreinforcing environment.

In the first situation, the dayroom is the reinforcer; in the second situation, the health provider is the reinforcer. As noted before, time-out means time out from positive reinforcement; therefore it is important to accurately identify all positive reinforcers before initiating this procedure. Since time-out serves as a form of punishment, it is important to consider more positive approaches or reductive procedures before using time-out. Once it has been decided to use time-out, all health providers should be trained in specific techniques for using the procedure accurately and effectively.

Reducing Behavior: Response Cost—An Aversive Approach

What follows are examples of response cost, an aversive technique for reducing undesirable behavior.

BEHAVIOR	CONSEQUENCE
Speeding ------------------------------>	$40.00 fine
Late for work -------------------------->	Loss in salary
Fighting ------------------------------->	Loss of phone privileges
Refusing to bathe ---------------------->	Loss of extra afternoon snack

Definition of Response Cost:
Response cost is "a reductive procedure in which a specific amount of available positive reinforcers are contingently withdrawn following the response" (Sulzer-Azaroff and Mayer, 1977:522).

Although response cost is minimally intrusive, it still remains an aversive procedure, and as such it may generate escape or aggressive behavior. As with other aversive procedures, ethical and legal issues must be considered. Response cost is a procedure that may be used to temporarily reduce undesirable behavior while alternative behaviors are being strengthened. When combined with positive reinforcement for desirable behaviors, response cost can lead to dramatic results.

Increasing Behavior: Escape—An Aversive Approach

The dialogues that follow demonstrate escape behavior. In each case, note the provider's response to the client's repeated requests.

Client: "Can I have a cigarette now? Oh, please can I have one now? Just this one time?"

Provider: "Oh, all right, here's your cigarette."

Client: "Is it time for my bath?"

Provider: "No. Your bath is scheduled in a half hour."

Client: "Can't I take my bath now? Can't I just start my bath?"

Provider: "Oh, OK, I'll run your water early just this once."

Giving the client the cigarette and running the bath water helped the provider escape from aversive nagging. In both cases, the behavior of "giving in" has been strengthened because it turned off something aversive—the nagging. Escape behavior and avoidance together comprise what is called *negative reinforcement.*

Definition of Escape Behavior:
Escape behavior occurs when a person attempts to end or terminate exposure to an aversive object or event, known as a stimulus (Mertens, 1982:144).

Escape behaviors are an everyday occurrence (e.g., moving away from a hot fire, turning off a loud alarm clock, coming in out of the cold, taking a verbal response "back," hallucinating if a problem cannot be handled, and responding to persistent questions). There is one "catch." With the principle of escape, escaping from something aversive may actually reinforce undesirable behavior. In the previous provider/client scenarios, the health provider has escaped from the nagging. However, in doing so, the provider has actually reinforced (by giving in) the very behaviors that were bothersome. The provider has temporarily escaped from the aversive behavior; however, the client has learned, "If I keep nagging long enough, I can get my way." Eliminating problem behaviors maintained by negative reinforcement can be accomplished by combining extinction with reinforcement for alternative positive behaviors.

CRITERIA FOR DEVELOPING A BEHAVIOR PROGRAM

Ogden Lindsley has developed an easily learned format for modifying behavior (Mertens, 1981:86). Lindsley outlines his technique with the following key steps:

1. Pinpoint the target behavior.
2. Count the responses.
3. Introduce a consequence immediately after the behavior.
4. Try, try again.

Pinpoint. The first step is to pinpoint the behavior to be changed, the target behavior. This behavior must be defined in terms that are specific, identifiable, and as precise as possible. It would not be very useful, for example, to state the goal as "improve grooming skills." "Improve" must be defined more precisely. One way to do this is to ask, "What is it the person must do?" A possible answer to this question might be: "He is to shave his entire face and comb his hair each morning before breakfast." In the latter statement, the behavior is defined in specific terms that can now be measured in order to determine changes in behavior.

Count (or record). The second step is to count and record the actual number of times a given behavior occurs before initiating any intervention. This base rate, or starting level of behavior, is very important. Using the previous example, if baseline data showed the client had a frequency of shaving 50 per cent of his face 3 days out of 7 days and combing his hair 3 days out of 7 days, this information could then serve as a standard against which the program approach would be compared. Baseline data, as well as data recorded daily, make it possible to objectively determine whether the consequence that immediately followed the behavior changed that behavior.

Introduce a consequence. Introducing a consequence immediately after the behavior involves trying to determine what consequence might influence the person's behavior, then presenting it to the person contingent on his performance of the desired behavior. Daily charting of the behavior provides continuous feedback as to the effectiveness of the reinforcement procedure.

Try, try, again. If after careful daily recording it is found during evaluation that the consequence has not changed the behavior, the data then indicate that it is time to try another consequence. As mentioned in the introduction to this section, applied behavior analysis is an ongoing process of analyzing and re-analyzing goals and the methods used to obtain those goals.

CRITERIA FOR EVALUATING
A BEHAVIOR PROGRAM

The following criteria have been designed to assist the health provider in spotting possible problems in a behavior program. They can be used as a checklist when developing a program and as a means to evaluate an existing program:

1. Was the behavior to be changed (target behavior) clearly specified?
2. Did the program provide for immediate reinforcement?
3. Did it outline small steps to attain the desired behavior?
4. Did reinforcement occur frequently and in small amounts?
5. Did the program call for and reinforce accomplishment rather than obedience?
6. Was the performance of the desired behavior reinforced **after** its occurrence?
7. Was the program for changing or modifying the behavior positive?
8. Was the program for changing or modifying the behavior mutually negotiated, if possible?

In summary, one of the greatest advantages to using behavior change techniques is the results that occur. Clearly identifiable changes in behavior can be accomplished using the principles described in this section.

REFERENCES

Hall, R.V., 1971. Managing Behavior: Application in School and Home. Lawrence, Kansas, H & H Enterprises.

Panyan, M.C., 1972. Managing Behavior. Lawrence, Kansas, H&H Enterprises.

Mertens, G., 1981. Behavioral Science Behaviorally Taught. Lexington, Mass, Ginn Custom.

Mertens, G., O'Brien, S., Lamberg, P., and Larsen, S., 1982. Workbook for Behavioral Science Behaviorally Taught: A Personalized Text for Learning About a Science of Behavior. Lexington, Mass, Ginn Custom.

O'Leary, K.D., and Wilson, G.T., 1975. Behavior Therapy: Application and Outcome. Englewood Cliffs, N.J., Prentice-Hall.

Schaefer, H.H., and Marten, P.L., 1967. Behavioral Therapy. New York, McGraw-Hill.

Silverman, M., 1980. How to Handle Problem Behaviors in School. Lawrence, Kansas, H&H Enterprises.

Singer, J.L., 1974. Imagery and Daydream Methods in Psychotherapy and Behavior Modification. New York, Academic Press.

Skinner, B.S., 1974. About Behaviorism. New York, Alfred A. Knopf.

Skinner, B.S., 1953. Science in Human Behavior. New York, Macmillan.

Sulzer-Azaroff, B., and Mayer, G., 1977. Applying Behavioral Analysis Procedures with Children and Youth. New York, Holt, Rinehart and Winston.

ACTIVITY THERAPY

LEARNING OBJECTIVES—Upon completing this chapter, the reader will be able to:

1. Describe the function of activity therapy.
2. Give five basic goals of therapeutic recreation.
3. Explain the purpose of work therapy.

Activities are a significant part of the developmental process. They provide a link between one's inner self and the external world. It is through activities that one learns about the world, tests knowledge, practices skills, expresses feelings, experiences pleasure, develops competence, and achieves mastery over one's life (Hopkins and Smith, 1978: 298). All of these functions of activities provide an outlet for the continuous flow of energy. Emotional problems can inhibit or block this natural outlet for energy; therefore, in working with persons who have emotional or psychiatric problems, it is important to include specific activities in their plan of care. Activities that are planned for a specific purpose or, in other words, that are goal-directed comprise activity therapy.

Activity therapy is a collective term used in many psychiatric settings to include therapeutic recreation, occupational therapy, play therapy, music therapy, dance therapy, art therapy, and work therapy (Avedon, 1974:38). In this section, only activity therapy in the broad sense, with a special focus on therapeutic recreation and work therapy, will be discussed. "Activity therapy is used to promote recovery through the release of excess energy and prevention of regression; the provision of a vehicle for self-expression; the practice of social skills in a protected, accepting environment; the acquisition of new knowledge; the development of new technical and creative skills; the correction of physical and psychological impairment; the achievement of self-actualization and the development of a sense of responsibility" (Kreigh and Perko, 1983:407).

In order that the activity be directed toward meeting the specific need of the client for whom it is prescribed or recommended, it is necessary to assess the client's emotional and physical needs and his strengths and weaknesses. The knowledge of strengths, which might include old interests and successes, can be used to help the client cope with his present situation and develop new interests. After the initial assessment, which provides baseline data, an activity therapy program can be planned for the individual client. The following are some guidelines to follow in planning an activity therapy program:

1. The activity should be in keeping with the client's lifestyle.
2. The activity should be of interest to the client.
3. The activity should utilize the client's strengths and abilities.
4. The activity should be short enough that the client feels he has accomplished something.
5. The activity should provide some new experiences for the client.
6. The client should be involved as much as possible in selecting the activity.

7. The client should receive only the help that is necessary to perform the activity.

8. The selected activity should be the client's, not the health provider's (Irving, 1983: 95–96).

Activity therapy is a very important part of the client's treatment program; therefore, it is crucial that the health provider become involved in his client's activity program. This involvement includes participating with the specialists who are providing the activity and following through on their recommendations to ensure continuity of care for the client.

THERAPEUTIC RECREATION

Therapeutic recreation enables persons with limitations to engage in recreational experiences. Some underlying principles of therapeutic recreation are (1) that everyone is responsible for meeting his own need for recreation experience; and (2) that the recreation experience is individualized to meet the client's specific needs in regard to his physical capability, availability, cost factor, and the continuation of the activity in the community. Therefore, "one cannot 'legislate' recreative experience per se, and . . . it is impossible to say, 'Come to the recreation room and be recreated'" (Avedon, 1974:25). Complaints from clients in residential institutions that there is nothing to do on weekends or in the evenings are evidence that "they [the clients] are unaware of their own potential for doing something about the recreation problems and the boredom they face" (Avedon. 25).

An area that is stressed under therapeutic recreation is leisure counseling. The content of classes on the effective use of leisure time focuses on recreational activities that can be performed throughout the life span, such as golf, swimming, running or jogging, and chess, rather than basketball, football, and other activities that are performed during a limited period of life and that require other persons' involvement. The activities are designed to help meet the client's maximum potential and functioning during leisure time.

A therapeutic recreational specialist is an asset to the health care team. Since the recreational specialist focuses on the healthy aspects of the client's personality, he observes the client's unusual behavior responses to popular recreational activities and reports the data to the health care team. The therapeutic recreational specialist teaches, guides, and leads recreational activity that is therapeutic by its very nature and make-up.

Some basic goals for a therapeutic recreation program are:

1. To provide a nonthreatening and nondemanding environment for the client. A client may refuse to participate in a recreational activity because he fears he cannot do it.

2. To provide the client with activities that are relaxing and that don't have rigid guidelines and time frames.

3. To provide the client with activities that will be enjoyable and self-satisfying.

4. To encourage the client's social interaction and help decrease his fear of contacting other persons.

5. To decrease the client's withdrawal tendencies.

6. To provide outlets for the client's excess energy, physical tension, and negative feelings.

7. To promote the client's socially acceptable behavior.

8. To develop the client's skills, talents, and abilities so that he can assume responsibility for his own recreation and use these techniques as alternative ways of dealing with problems he thought were insoluble.

9. To increase the client's self-confidence and feeling of self-worth.

10. To revitalize the client's physical strength and mental awareness.

11. To provide for continuity of recreational activities in the community so that clients will be able to meet their needs upon discharge (Quigley and Walcott, 1972:56).

12. To provide a reality focus that is productive and constructive.

WORK THERAPY*

Because work provides a common status and position in the community, it draws people together. According to Levinson (1964:2, 11), "work is a psychological glue which often holds a man together. . . . Work heals by a number of mechanisms. Work imposes structure on time when a person might otherwise be unable to self-impose organization. Work provides tasks and goals when depression might otherwise lead a person to feel worthless. Work results in productivity and productivity conveys a sense of self-worth and self-dignity." In addition, a by-product of work is earned income. Money provides everyone with an access to power, achievement, success, safety, and public recognition. The unemployed tend to lose their motivation to solve their problems and may appear to have lost their skill and confidence in coping with reality.

It has been estimated that approximately 80 per cent of patients admitted to state mental hospitals can be helped through alternative forms of psychiatric care without the need for hospitalization or at least with only a short period of inpatient care (Black, 1977:32–33). Some facilities are able to provide a place in which activity therapies, training activities of daily living, prevocational services, and sheltered work activities prepare the client to work in his home community. One of the most difficult population groups to work with in a mental health setting is the chronically mentally ill who experience repeated hospitalizations. These clients often display symptoms such as bizarre behavior, hallucinations, delusions, or severe withdrawal. Health providers initially may have to supervise routine behaviors, such as sleep and rest, grooming and hygiene, nutrition and elimination. As the client gradually assumes more responsibility for his actions and achievements, he develops pride in himself for what he can accomplish. Dowd and Dowd stated that through environmental manipulation and medication, stress and ambiguity may be reduced for the client with schizophrenia. In addition, use of supportive therapy, such as focusing on coping and maintenance skills, can prevent further deterioration. The client with depression may be helped through an increase in meaningful activity that will heighten his self-esteem, personal reinforcement, and sense of purpose, while diminishing his sense of loss (Dowd and Dowd, 1981:41). Activities that are meaningful to the client must be stressed, since often clients with mental illness are placed in activities/programs because health providers decide that the activity or program will help them. Placing the client in activities that are meaningless to him expends needless time and energy for both client and health provider. The key, then, is to find an environment in which the client will be motivated to work.

In working with the organically impaired client, a structured, nonthreatening, mildly stimulating, basic routine is essential. Ideas should be presented to the client in a supportive and exploratory manner to draw the client out, rather than in a directive manner that may further push him into his world of self-containment (Dowd and Dowd, 1981:40).

Health providers often ask themselves if it is worth the time and effort to involve their clients in a rehabilitation program if employers are not going to employ them. Those familiar with vocational rehabilitation realize that it is every rehabilitation facility's goal to place clients in the optimum working environment. Should the optimum working

---

*This section was written by Michael Hill, M.S.

environment be competitive employment, then this becomes the goal, again with the idea of securing a job that is meaningful to the client.

Clients are affected by long periods of inactivity, which allows them time to dwell on concerns of returning to work. Amdur and Amdur (1984:16) stated that not working for a period of time can be distressing to the client and can additionally increase the stigma and social distance the client feels about returning to work. In addition, time off from work increases a client's concern about being able to return to his former job and of the job's availability, particularly after a lengthy absence. The decision to return the client to a vocational setting is the result of a health team decision that includes the client. The following questions are helpful in making this decision:

1.   Can the client handle the stress of a work setting caused by factors such as interactions with co-workers, working a specified number of hours, and following simple instructions? Clients who hear voices can learn to ignore the voices and continue to perform the work task.

2.   Has the client displayed appropriate judgment with regard to personal safety and medication?

3.   Has the client displayed appropriate grooming and hygiene?

Once these questions have been answered, the next step is to determine the client's replacement into the vocational setting through the possible restructuring of his duties and hours. Another possibility is placement in an alternative vocational setting through the use of volunteer work.

The client should be gradually reintroduced into a vocational setting to reduce the shock of transition from hospital to work. To facilitate this, health providers should know what the employer can offer regarding work positions, time expectations, and production standards. According to Amdur and Amdur (1984:16), when a health provider, such as a psychiatrist, indicates that the client should return to work in a less stressful capacity, the specific number of work hours, the amount of interpersonal contact, the production demands, and the amount of supervision needed should be defined.

Another possible avenue to pursue with the client is to seek out volunteer work. Volunteer work should not be minimized just because the client is not earning income, since the activity in itself is important. At this point, volunteer work provides two opportunities for the client. First, meaningful volunteer work can be used as a stepping stone to competitive work, since it provides all the components of competitive work, but with less stress. Often, the work hours and days are more flexible, and self-confidence can be gradually regained. The second benefit of volunteer work is perhaps more applicable to the client with chronic mental difficulties who may never work. As previously mentioned, meaningful activity, including volunteer work, can be beneficial because it provides an active way of stimulating the client, as opposed to allowing the client to do nothing and to dwell on his problems.

A question that often arises is whether the employer should be told that the client has had mental illness. The Affirmative Action Program states that an employer cannot refuse to consider a client for work because the client has had a mental illness unless the illness would impair the client's ability to do a specific job (DHHS 81-1073, 1981:10). It is recommended that the client write in "will explain" where the application asks about mental illness. When the client meets with the employer, he can explain that for a period of time he was experiencing difficulty but has been working to get his life in order. He may go on to discuss his job skills and accomplishments.

Often the client's job performance is very good; it is the loneliness after work that tends to pull the client down. The client needs to get involved in activities outside of work, such as church groups, mental health support groups, Y.M.C.A., and bowling leagues.

TABLE 15-1. Suggested Activities, Recreation, and Work for Specific Patterns of Behavior

PATTERNS OF BEHAVIOR	ACTIVITIES	RECREATION	WORK
Anxious behavior characterized by nervousness, helplessness, complaining, crying, irritability, demanding of time and attention, and somatic complaints, such as chest pains, heart palpitations, sweating, insomnia, loss of appetite, and gastrointestinal distress	—Simple concrete task or simple game —Painting —Gardening —Any activity that will get individual outside himself	—Walking (Allow client to pace.) —Body contact sports (for aggressive urges) —Jogging —Active, physical, aerobic activity	—Simple tasks with no more than three to four steps that can be learned quickly. For example: —Kitchen tasks, such as clearing and washing tables —Sweeping or mopping floors —Outdoor work such as mowing lawn and weeding flowers —The client's expression of boredom may signal his readiness for more complex tasks.
Withdrawal behavior characterized by loss of contact with reality and little or no interest in the world around him; fear; staring into space; hearing voices; disorganized thinking; and impulsive behavior	—Simple, concrete tasks in which client is actively involved, such as: —Metal work and modeling clay (uses touch; chance to be creative) —Social activities to give client contact with others and reality —Activity of daily living skills	—Dancing —Noncompetitive athletics —Outings (e.g., picnics) —Hobby discussion groups	—Simple work goals in 15- to 30-minute blocks of time. At the end of each block of time, praise for goals achieved and encourage appropriately. —If client is hearing voices or otherwise losing touch with reality, interrupt process and reinforce reality. —Client needs continuous supervision and at first works best on a one-to-one basis.
Overly suspicious behavior characterized by mistrust, hostility, irritability, fears of persecution, impulsive and destructive behavior, misinterpretation of actions, refusal of food and medications on basis of being poisoned, and blaming others for own discomforts.	—Noncompetitive, solitary, meaningful tasks that require some degree of concentration, such as jigsaw puzzles, crossword puzzles, scrabble, leather tooling, and ceramics. Through concentration, less time is available for focusing on delusions; activities use small and large muscles and cognitive functions (Payne and Clunn, 1977:96).	—Avoid competitive, aggressive activities that involve close contact. —Provide outlets for anger, aggressive drives. —Client will experience success in groups when trust is established.	—Solitary occupations (e.g., interior decorating); client needs to organize and receive positive feedback. —A task that requires concentration is desirable. After skill and confidence are gained, have client work with another client as a task trainer. Develop a buddy system.
Depressed behavior characterized by hopelessness, helplessness, sadness, low self-esteem, worthlessness, fatigue, sleep disturbances, loss of appetite, weight loss, and preoccupation with death.	—Simple tasks that can be finished, such as pouring a ceramic mold (client needs to experience success) —Activities of daily living (use simple but structured schedule)	—Noncompetitive team sports (provide outlets for anger; use up energy) —Jogging, running or walking briskly —Achievement- and success-oriented activity, such as crafts, hobbies, service to others	—Tasks that are helpful; such as folding laundry, cleaning ashtrays, emptying wastebaskets (client feels more worthy when a needed job is done.) —Challenge client to complete one more task within a specific period of time. Offer positive reinforcement after each achievement.
Overactive (manic) behavior characterized by hyperactivity; short attention span with flight of ideas; aggressiveness; domineering and meddlesome behavior; playing staff members against each other; little attention to physical needs; low frustration level that may lead to destructiveness, defective judgment, and sarcasm.	—Noncompetitive activities that allow the use of energy and expression of feelings (e.g., tearing rags, writing and drawing, pounding on a leather belt). Such activities should be *limited* and *changed frequently.* —Things that are simple and quickly done —Activities of daily living (e.g., personal grooming)	—Ball, badminton on one-to-one basis, (for short periods of time) —Individual games that are physical and active	—Housekeeping tasks —Raking grass (large sweeping movements are good) —It is helpful to have client work in an area away from distractions, such as people walking through. —Use work goals interchangeably with the amount of money earned. For example, the more you accomplish the more money you earn.

Table continues on following page.

TABLE 15–1. Suggested Activities, Recreation, and Work for Specific Patterns of Behavior
(Continued)

PATTERNS OF BEHAVIOR	ACTIVITIES	RECREATION	WORK
Emotionally disturbed child/adolescent characterized by ceaseless activity; quarrelsome, defiant behavior that interferes with client's relationships at home and school	*Child:* Play that is fun and recreational, such as: —story telling —painting —poetry or music *Adolescent:* Creative activities, such as: —leather work —painting —sculpture (Payne and Clunn, 1977:118, 127)	*Child:* —Better to work with child on a one-to-one basis. Give child a feeling of importance; put him in a role of leadership and assistance. Establish a positive relationship with child. *Adolescent:* —Does better in groups —Gross motor activity to use up excess energy (e.g., sports, games)	—If old enough to work, the adolescent does best as an assistant to an adult worker. —Reinforce him no matter how small the achievement is. —Work suggestions include: —Auto repair —Kitchen work —Feeding clients —Making beds
Acting out behavior characterized by charming, intelligent, but superficial, inconsistent, and untruthful behavior. Knows what is right and wrong, but does what is easiest at the moment. Does not learn from experience; shows poor judgment, manipulates others, and is source of much friction	—Activities that enhance self-esteem and are expressive and creative but not too complicated, for example, making posters for a dance. (This client tends to offer to do numerous tasks without following through; client needs supervision to make sure each task is completed.)	—Cooking —Jogging —Service groups and projects for others	—Initially place clients away from other clients if seen as a source of distraction or friction. —Praise work that is well done. Have client redo poor work. Supervise closely to be sure tasks are completed. —Have client start with simple, boring tasks; progress to more difficult and interesting tasks. If acting out occurs, have client work on boring task. As behavior improves, again place him on more difficult, interesting task as reward for desired behavior.
Organic brain impairment characterized by poor judgment; labile affect; poor memory (loss of recent events; remembers remote events); confusion; disorientation to time, place, and person	—Group activities to increase feelings of belonging and self-worth. —Promote familiar, individual hobbies. Activities need to be structured, requiring little time for completion and not much concentration. —Reality orientation as to time, place, and, if necessary, person. —Reminiscent or life review activities.	—Concrete, repetitious crafts and projects that breed familiarization and comfort.	—Choose a task that builds upon itself after a period of time. During the first part of the task, explain and demonstrate how the procedure should be done. Then have client repeat the demonstration. This step may have to be repeated daily, for several days, depending on the client. —Some clients will have to continue with the basic task indefinitely.
Alcoholism characterized by drinking excessively when one does not mean to, such as first thing in the morning; low frustration level; dependency; shakiness; insecurity; hostility; making demands; lack of self-respect; guilty feelings; denying or minimizing drinking; and manipulativeness.	—Group activities in which client uses his talents and assets. For example, involve client in planning social activities; encourage interaction with others.	—Leisure counseling (i.e., planned recreation for free time) —Leisure value clarification —Introduction to and participation in recreational activities as an alternative to substance abuse —Encourage responsibility for recreational activities.	—Insist that client complete work assignments. —Place on simple but meaningful work projects. A buddy system with another client who is displaying good work behaviors is effective. Work behaviors gradually change and friendships are developed. Any area of work can be appropriate. How the work is presented to the client is more significant than what the work actually is.

TABLE 15–1. Suggested Activities, Recreation, and Work for Specific Patterns of Behavior
(Continued)

PATTERNS OF BEHAVIOR	ACTIVITIES	RECREATION	WORK
Mental retardation and emotional disturbance characterized by a decrease in intellectual functioning with outbursts of temper.	—Simple activities at level of individual's functioning; break activities into small steps with positive reinforcement after accomplishing each step. This is helpful in teaching self-help skills, such as eating, dressing, brushing teeth. —Use adult pictures for coloring activity with adults.	—Recreational activities must be manipulated and adapted to fit level of client's functioning.	—Repetitive work assignments are ideal, since these clients do not get bored. This type of work assignment is available in sheltered workshops. For example, subcontracting work, such as: —Capsuling —Making hammocks, bicycle brakes —Unwrapping cheese —Repackaging goods In all of these jobs, the client can experience success and be rewarded financially.

Like everyone else, the client benefits from social contacts; if he does not make contacts, he thinks only about his loneliness and problems. Social interactions, combined with a supportive therapeutic and vocational environment, will facilitate the client's replacement in the community.

Table 15–1 gives suggested activities, recreation, and work for specific patterns of behavior.

REFERENCES

Affirmative Action to Employ Mentally Restored People. DHHS publication 81-1073. U.S. Department of Health and Human Services, U.S. Department of Labor, pp. 1–17.

Amdur, M., and Amdur, M., 1984. The return of the mentally restored worker. NAP Digest, May/June, pp. 14–18.

Avedon, E.M., 1974. Therapeutic Recreation Service: An Applied Behavioral Science Approach. Englewood Cliffs, N.J., Prentice-Hall.

Beard, M.T., Enlow, C.T., and Owens, J.G., 1978. Activity therapy as a reconstructive plan on the social competence of chronic hospitalized patients. J Psychosoc Nurs Ment Health Serv, February, pp. 33–41.

Black, B.J., 1977. Substitute permanent employment for the deinstitutionalized mentally ill. J Rehabil, May/June, pp. 32–39.

Bragman, R., and Cole, J.C., 1983. Perceived differences in the job potential of individuals with visible and nonvisible disabilities. J Rehabil, October/November/December, pp. 47–51.

Dowd, T., and Dowd, T., 1981. Rehabilitation of mentally ill older adults. J Rehabil, October/November/December, pp. 38–41.

Dunlop, L., 1978. Conducting a therapeutic community. In Mental Health Concepts Applied to Nursing, New York, Wiley.

Hopkins, M.A., and Smith, H.D. (eds.), 1978. Willard and Spackman's Occupational Therapy, 5th ed. Philadelphia, J.B. Lippincott.

Knowles, R., 1981. Handling depression through activity. Am J Nurs, Vol. 81, No. 6, p. 1187.

Kreigh, H., and Perko, J., 1983. Psychiatric and Mental Health Nursing: A Commitment to Care and Concern. Reston, Va.; Reston Publishing.

Lancaster, J., 1975. Activity groups as therapy. Am J Nurs, Vol. 76, No. 6, pp. 947–949.

Levinson, H., 1964. What work means to a man. Menninger Q, Summer/Autumn, Vol. 18, No. 213, pp. 1–11.

People with chronic schizophrenia: Their rehabilitation outlook. 1983 Rehabil Brief, Vol. 6, No. 2, pp. 1–4.

Quigley, J., and Walcott, A., 1972. Recreation renews interest in life. Hospitals, November 1, Vol. 46, pp. 53–57.

Spooner, F., Alzozzine, B., and Saxon, J., 1980. The efficiency of vocational rehabilitation with mentally ill persons. J Rehabil, October/November/December, pp. 62–66.

USE OF RELAXATION, IMAGERY, TOUCH, AND HUMOR

LEARNING OBJECTIVES—Upon completing this chapter, the reader will be able to:

1. Describe the relaxation methods of Roon, Benson, and Jacobson.

2. Outline the use of imagery with a client experiencing anger.

3. List five ways of using touch in establishing contact with a client.

4. Give two positive uses of humor as it relates to the communication process.

USE OF RELAXATION

In any setting, the health provider is faced with clients who feel overwhelmed by their response to stressful situations in their life. A provider can do more than just empathize with the client if he has learned some relaxation techniques that can be modified to meet the needs of the particular client. "All living things are constantly under stress, and anything—pleasant or unpleasant—that speeds up the intensity of life causes a temporary increase in stress, the wear and tear exerted on the body. A painful blow and a passionate kiss can be equally as stressful" (Selye, 1965:97). It is, in other words, our *reaction* to a situation, rather than the situation itself, that causes stress. Individuals seem to do best with a moderate amount of stress in their lives. "High stress is accompanied by high levels of adrenaline in the body, but studies show that if people are bored and understimulated, their adrenaline levels are also high. If they are moderately stimulated the levels are lower" (Bolysenko, 1984:69). What constitutes moderate stress stimulation varies greatly from person to person. The health provider must keep this in mind as he teaches clients to manage stressful situations in their lives wisely.

Relaxation training is one way to manage stress. During a relaxed state, the heart slows down, the respiratory rate falls, the metabolism rate and blood pressure are lowered, and muscular tension is decreased. Along with the physical responses to relaxation, the client also experiences a sense of well-being. As the mind and body become calm, the client feels refreshed and revitalized. "Studies show that people who practice daily relaxation react quicker to stressors, and recover more quickly than those who do not practice relaxation" (Schiralde, 1982:10). Before considering relaxation training for the client, the health provider must know some basic information. Most important is that relaxation training is not for everyone. Occasionally, the health provider is tempted to assume that a technique that is suitable for him will surely be the answer for others as well. Tuttle (1982:81) lists cautions for relaxation, and notes that "approximately 3% of patients respond to relaxation training by actually increasing arousal (e.g., increasing blood pressure instead of decreasing)." He further notes that most medications (including medication for diabetes, epilepsy, and thyroid replacement) become more potent during relaxation, and, consequently, the client requires medical monitoring. Individuals with hypertension or glaucoma can have a recurrence of illness without knowing it. Clients over 65 years of age with hypotension are also poor candidates for relaxation training. Clients on large doses of narcotics or anti-anxiety medications may need to have their medication reduced or eliminated while engaged in relaxation training. Finally, Tuttle, along with other researchers, has found that clients who are experiencing psychoses do not respond positively to relaxation training.

Many relaxation methods are available, and it follows that the method taught must be tailored to the client's lifestyle. This is important because the long-term goal is to have the client manage his own stress on a day-to-day basis. The object is to provide a tool that will induce relaxation but will not cause the client to fall asleep, unless this is the purpose of the relaxation.

The following guidelines may be helpful in deciding with the client what his needs are and which relaxation method is best suited to meet his needs:

1.   Obtain a data base. Have the client record all high levels of stress for two or three days to help assess the stress pattern. The following format is suggested:

DATE TIME	INCIDENT	OUTCOME	WHAT HAPPENED PRIOR TO INCIDENT

2.   Explore with the client previous positive ways of dealing with stress. If possible, incorporate some of this information into a relaxation plan for the client. Remember that neither recreation nor sleep is synonymous with relaxation.

3.   Ask the client how he visualizes relaxation occurring (i.e., head to toe or vice versa). If the client needs to learn progressive relaxation, determine the order of relaxation according to this information.

4.   Decide on a regular practice time. Some clients will want to start their day with a relaxation exercise. Some clients will want to end their day in this way. Short, on-the-spot relaxation exercises can be utilized as needed throughout the day. Overall relaxation training is accomplished most readily before meals or at least two hours after a meal because of the stimulant effect of food on the body. Caffeine-containing drinks, such as regular coffee and some soft drinks, are best avoided prior to the training session.

In a homogeneous group, it is often possible to simultaneously teach several clients with similar relaxation needs. Benson suggests four basic components necessary for eliciting a relaxation response, regardless of the method used (1976:159–161). The components are:

—A quiet environment
—A mental device
—A passive attitude
—A comfortable position

A quiet environment helps eliminate distractions and permits the client to concentrate on a mental device of his choosing. A mental device is any sound, word, or phrase that evokes a sense of calm. The client repeats the device silently or out loud with eyes closed. If the client prefers to keep his eyes open, he can fix his gaze upon an object. Either way, the client's mind is focused on one thing. Concentrating on his normal breathing pattern also enhances the client's repetition of the mental device. A passive attitude is considered most significant for eliciting a successful relaxation response. The client needs reassurance in advance that distracting thoughts may occur. Instruct the client to simply let the thoughts pass through and return to the repetition of the mental device. Relaxation is a learned skill, and, as Trygstad (1980:30) pointed out, ". . . relaxation is one of the few skills where 'trying hard' is actually a detriment as it usually creates tension." A comfortable position prevents additional muscular tension. Sitting with good posture, loose fitting clothes, shoes off, and feet on the floor is a preferred position. Lying down is not encouraged, since clients tend to fall asleep. The exception is for progressive relaxation and exercises used to promote rest and sleep.

Modules offered for relaxation training appear to be based on the work of a small number of major theorists. Table 16–1 presents relaxation methods based on the work of Roon, Benson, and Jacobson.

It is essential that the health provider first learn to relax himself before attempting to help the client relax. It is further recommended that the health provider practice each exercise completely, prior to introducing it to a client. An interesting paradox is involved in teaching relaxation to a client. "Each time you teach a patient to relax, you'll reduce the stress you live and work with, and improve your own sense of well being" (Trygstad, 1980: 32).

USE OF IMAGERY

Feelings and thoughts are pulled toward one's mental images, and the client, most often, becomes what he imagines he can become. The nervous system operates on imagery, and the client's personal images serve as a self-fulfilling prophecy. Images go directly to the nervous system. Consider the image produced by "blue Monday" and "Thank God it's Friday!" Each image sets the tone for the day. Images are used for or against oneself, and when one is tired the negative images seem to make the maximum impression. Similarly, clients who picture themselves as failing to deal with their problems of daily living are apt to end up with trouble. It is possible, with selected clients, to encourage them to think about a time when they may have operated successfully, even if only briefly, and to teach them how to change negative images into positive images of successful coping. Lazarus (1977:3–4) suggests that imagery can be used to overcome fear, anxiety, depression, anger, feelings of inferiority, and other negative emotions. It can also help counter bad habits, such as smoking and overeating; and enhance aspects of life, such as creativity at work, proficiency at sports, and general patterns of communication.

It is not the intent here to deal with guided imagery that requires a psychotherapist to guide and deal with symbolic material that may emerge as a result of the imagery (Leuner, 1969:4–22). Instead, our intent is to present imagery the client can learn to use as a way of moving through anxiety-provoking situations. Some clients will be better at imagining than others. Some may see only shadowy figures, while another sees vivid, technicolor images. Images need not be particularly vivid to be effective. Mental pictures do seem to come more easily when the client is relaxed and free of distraction. Consequently, after determining the goal with the client, the first step is to begin with a relaxation exercise suited to the client's needs. The second step is to follow with the imagery. Two or three breaths are helpful prior to the imagery; for example, Inhale—Exhale—Pause, then repeat. Additional progressive relaxation may be needed by a very tense client. At first, the health provider will have to guide the client through the relaxation and imagery to prevent the client from becoming side-tracked. When the human mind wanders, it focuses on negative, unfinished business. The health provider's guidance gently pulls the mind away from the negative thoughts to focus on the imagery. This is not to be interpreted as a form of repression but rather as a way of changing mental images that, in turn, influence the way the client feels about and responds behaviorally to a given situation. In practicing the imagery, it is important to take sufficient time to include enough detail to permit the client to "get into" the imagery. Conclude the imagery by bringing the client to an alert state. When he is ready, have him count from one to ten and continue to sit with his eyes closed. When he is ready, have him open his eyes and stretch. Have him continue sitting a while longer before getting up.

Table 16–2 includes just several of the many ways that imagery can be useful to a client.

Clients must be reminded that if they experience anxiety anytime during the imagery, they need only to open their eyes, look around, reorient themselves to their surroundings, and, when satisfied, close their eyes and continue with the imagery. Some clients are comfortable with their eyes open during the entire process and do not seem to have any problem visualizing the images suggested. Imagery, like other techniques, takes self-discipline; therefore, it is recommended that the health provider plan with the client for daily practice sessions. An evaluation of the effectiveness of this technique, which is most often evidenced by behavioral change, is an integral part of the health provider's responsibility to the client.

Not only is imagery a useful tool for better living for the client, but it can become a surprisingly easy way for the client to develop some sense of control over his response to problems of daily living. Lazarus also suggests that imagery can be used to protect against future shock, such as job losses, love losses, or marital problems, by visualizing the situation and potential outcome in advance. Imagery can also be fun and a creative way to pass the time. The health provider is reminded that each step leading to his career as health provider was preceded by first visualizing the steps and the possible outcome. "Visualization becomes real when the idea of 'creating one's own reality' through use of imagination becomes experience rather than theory" (Vissing and Burke, 1984:31).

USE OF TOUCH

Sometimes in the course of necessary care, touch is mechanical, a part of the job being done, and conveys no caring message. Some health providers use caring touch and are unaware of it. Touching involves risk. It may be misunderstood by both the client and the health provider. Since it involves intimate space, it may be a threat. If the health provider is not in tune with himself and is not sensitive as to how he comes across, his touch may seem inappropriate and offensive to the client. On the other hand, nontouch may be just as harmful. At times, words cannot reach the client, perhaps because of his inability to process information. The client may also hide his need for touch because he feels it is inappropriate or childish and will sometimes seek this closeness through sex. A careful look at the client's sexual activity may reveal that he was actually seeking physical closeness. "But touch is even more basic than sex as a primary drive" (Huss, 1977:14). It has even been suggested that perhaps one reason clients may turn to drugs is to compensate for the lack of touch in their lives, which is the first tranquilizer the child experiences.

Sometimes touch is withheld out of fear of having touch misinterpreted as a homosexual or heterosexual advance. Some clients make rules for themselves such as, "If I don't touch someone of the opposite or same sex, it will be O.K." Consequently, they lavish their need to touch on pets.

It has been suggested that the minimum daily requirement for hugs per day is 4; 8 hugs for a good day; and 12 for a great day (Risberg, 1984:Seminar). If this is considered the need for the mentally healthy person, what does it say about the need for hugs for the emotionally disturbed client?

"The need for body contact, which signifies being loved, comforted, accepted and protected can be affected by illness, anger, anxiety and depression" (Huss, 1977:15). The

TABLE 16-1. Relaxation Methods and Directions to Client

ORIGINATOR AND SYNOPSIS OF RELAXATION METHOD	DIRECTIONS TO CLIENT
ROON—Applied Relaxation	Part your lips slightly.
Brief relaxation. This exercise prevents rush of thought. It can be used to induce on-the-spot relaxation in a public place or to promote sleep.	Place the tip of the tongue behind the lower teeth. Keep it there without pressure for awhile. Continue with normal breathing.
Yawning. This is a one-minute tension-release exercise. The lungs expand; the back, jaw, mouth, and tongue relax. More oxygen comes into the system. Nice to do near an open window.	Drop your jaw gently until it feels large enough to take in a whole fruit. As you begin to yawn, it feels as though it will never end. As you yawn, you are taking in a deep breath. When the yawn ends, you feel relaxed, clear down into your stomach. Your lungs have expanded, and your back begins to release its tension.
Two-minute exercise. This exercise releases shoulder tension and is ideal for the client who will return to a job that requires hours of sitting.	Take a deep breath, hold it and raise your right shoulder. Gently roll it forward, up, back, and around in a complete circle. Exhale. Do the same thing with the left shoulder, always starting with a deep breath. Repeat for two minutes.
Five-minute relaxation. This exercise relaxes aching eyes, neck, and shoulders.	Close your eyes gently. Tell yourself that your eyes are dropping forward out of their sockets. You see nothing at all except soft, soothing darkness. Let your head drop until your jaw is almost on your chest; let the hinges of your jaw relax. Take a deep breath, and begin to rotate your head. Let it roll softly, first to the right, then to the left, then to the back, so it falls back on the shoulders. (That probably hurt a bit!) Then roll it to the left and forward. Now exhale and rest. Take a deep breath, and start to the left, rotating your head in the same way.
Five-minute rest period. This relaxation is ideal for the client returning to a situation where he will have limited time for himself.	Lie in a darkened room. Yawn deeply. Close your eyes and take a deep breath. Let your head drop limply. Part your lips slightly, relax your jaw. Smile to expand your nostrils. By breathing better, you are relaxing tension. Continue to breathe normally. When ready, open your eyes; get up slowly.
BENSON—Relaxation Response	
This easy-to-learn technique has four components: —A quiet environment —A mental device (a word, sound, phrase or gazing at an object) —A passive attitude —A comfortable position	Sit quietly in a comfortable position with your eyes closed (or open if gazing). Let your muscles relax, beginning at your feet and progressing up to your face. Breathe through your nose. As you breathe out, repeat a mental device (or continue to gaze at an object). For example: Breathe IN . . . OUT . . . (mental device). Eyes may be opened as desired to check the time. Simply close your eyes when satisfied, and return to repeating the mental device. Do not worry about being successful. Let distracting thoughts pass through. Simply return to repeating the mental device IN . . . OUT . . . (mental device). IN . . . OUT . . . (mental device).
Practice once or twice daily for 10 to 20 minutes. Gradually work up to 20 minutes once or twice daily.	When you desire to stop, sit quietly for several minutes, at first with eyes closed, then with the eyes open. Continue to sit for a few minutes; then get up slowly.
JACOBSON—Progressive Relaxation	*Introductory exercise*
This exercise is useful for the very tense client. The health provider directs him in relaxing skeletal	Have the client sit in a chair, close his eyes, and

TABLE 16-1. Relaxation Methods and Directions to Client—(Continued)

Originator and Synopsis of Relaxation Method	Directions to Client
muscles. This is a rather strenuous exercise and is best suited for someone in fairly good physical condition. Training is usually a half-hour to an hour, three to four times a week. The client is also encouraged to practice on his own. At no time does the health provider tell the client to stop thinking or to make his mind a blank. Directions include: 1. How to tense the various muscle groups 2. A reminder to be aware of the tension in each part of the body 3. Direction to relax and to note the difference. Demonstrate to the client how to relax and contract a muscle before beginning the exercise. An introductory exercise that teaches the client to recognize muscular tension is useful. No relaxing is attempted at this time.	explore areas of tension in his body without attempting to relax. The following order is suggested: —Left arm —Right arm —Left foot, leg, and thigh —Abdominal muscles —Chest muscles —Back and spine —Shoulder muscles that move the shoulders forward —Shoulder muscles that move the shoulders inward —Shoulder muscles used in shrugging —Muscles used in bending the head to the right, to the left, holding it stiffly —Muscles for wrinkling the brow —Frowning —Closing eyelids tightly —With eyelids closed lightly, looking to the left, right, up, down and forward —Smiling, rounding the lips to an "O," sticking the tongue out and putting it back in —Muscles used for closing the jaws tightly —Counting one to ten —Swallowing
Ask the client what areas he noted as being tense. Both the right and left sides may be relaxed at the same time. If the client is very tense, do one side at a time, beginning with the left. Space directions for the relaxation exercise so that the client tenses each muscle group for about 30 seconds, then relaxes the muscle group for about 60 seconds in order to experience the difference. Tell the client that different body sensations may be experienced as the body relaxes. Sensations of warmth, tingling, unusual heaviness or lightness are not unusual. Should the client feel uncomfortable, he can open his eyes, look around, and resume relaxing.	*Relaxation Exercise* Lie down with eyes closed, arms at the side, legs uncrossed. Take two or three deep breaths. Breathe deeply enough so that the abdomen rises while inhaling. For example: INHALE . . . EXHALE . . . Concentrate on your breathing for awhile, and continue to breathe naturally throughout the exercise. Tense each of the muscle groups as directed. Note the tension. Relax when the word *RELAX* is said and note the difference. *Ready?* —Point the feet and toes down. (Note the areas of tension. Relax. Note the difference.) —Point the toes up. —Straighten your legs out, and lock the knees. —Dig your heels into the floor. —Tense the groin and buttocks muscles at the same time. —Pull in the muscles of your stomach. —Push your shoulders down. Keep your buttocks down, and bring your chin to your chest. —Press your arms against your body. —Shrug your shoulders. —Bend your wrists up. —Make a fist. —Turn your head to the left. —Turn your head to the right. —Bring your chin to your chest. —Smile. Make a tight "O" with your lips. —Close your jaw tightly. —Stick your tongue way out. —Frown and shut your eyes tightly. —Raise your eyebrows.
The order of relaxation may be reversed to meet individual client's needs.	Continue to breathe normally. Stay with the feeling. When you are ready to return to an alert state, count slowly from one to ten. Open your eyes when you are ready.

TABLE 16–2. Imagery as a Way of Dealing with Specific Situations

Situation	Imagery
Anger	There is some concern that venting anger in fantasy may provide a rehearsal for actual aggressiveness (Berkowitz, 1971:24–31). Suggest that the client visualize the situation that helped create the angry feelings. Tell him to see himself as calm and in control, being able to get through the anger in a constructive way. Since anger often dies of neglect if it is not nurtured, the following new scripts are suggested as appropriate for the client to rehearse as he visualizes the original situation with a variety of different responses. Choose the appropriate scripts. Rehearse it many times. —I do not like it when you treat me this way. —This problem does not belong to me, and I do not have to feel angry just because you do. —I have other alternatives. I do not have to stay in this situation that frequently leaves me so angry. —I am clear-headed and intelligent. I am not going to fall apart and do something I will regret. —What am I doing to keep myself hooked into anger? —What am I getting out of being angry?
Anxiety	Have the client design his own favorite scene and see himself there, appropriately dressed (e.g., swimsuit, etc.) Have him take time to look around and visualize his surroundings with great detail. Suggest that he use all his senses to experience the sight, sound, smell, touch, and taste available in his special hideaway. Have him stay there for awhile and experience himself as peaceful and calm. Remind him that it is a safe place, and he can return there daily to rest. When he is ready to leave, have him take one look back, knowing that he can return any time. Tell him that he will continue to feel happy, relaxed, and peaceful as he returns to continue with his daily activities.
Interpersonal Relationships	Suggest that the client visualize the person involved and rehearse the meeting with this person. Have the client visualize the meeting in great detail: surroundings, clothing, etc. Imagine calmly speaking to and effectively answering questions presented by the person, even if he feels anxious inside. Have him visualize responding to both positive and negative statements, knowing that he will remain composed and confident. It is important to rehearse this scenario many times.
Sleeplessness	Have the client visualize a situation that he has experienced as boring or that he dislikes doing. Suggest that he recreate the scene in great detail, permitting himself to relive the sights, sounds, smells, etc., that were part of the original situation. Lazarus (1977:162) confides that visualizing a boring lecture that he has had to endure for at least three hours induces a deep, restful sleep for him in less than three minutes!
Work Skills	Have the client visualize awakening early enough to have time to groom appropriately. Have him imagine this preparation in detail. Have him visualize sitting down to his favorite breakfast, being aware of how it looks, tastes, and smells so good! Have him see himself leaving for work, energetic and ready, being aware of what his senses experience on the way. Have him repeat several times, "I am smart and capable. I will do my best. If I need help, I will ask for it." Have him visualize arriving at work; greeting other workers and the boss, if there; beginning work confidently and skillfully; knowing that if he needs help, he can ask for it without embarrassment. Have him see the boss come in to look at his work and hear him say, "That's a fine job you're doing!" Have him visualize also the boss saying, "Your work needs improvement." Then have him see himself remaining calm and saying to the boss, "I would appreciate some information on how to do this work better."

lack of touch and loneliness are thought to go together. Loneliness haunts the mentally ill, and loneliness is often described as the root of delusions. The client begins to fill his lonely time with fantasy. When there is insufficient human contact to balance the fantasy, the client may lose touch with what is real and what is fantasy.

Supporting the use of touch does not negate the importance of verbal communication. The health provider needs to recognize the need for a balance. Most health providers do not think of touch in a conscious manner and may not be aware of their feelings about being touched and touching, unless it has been brought to their attention. How, then, can health providers learn the use of touch and make it part of their daily contact with the client? The following suggestions are offered to the health provider:

1. Explore your own feelings about touch—your comfort level with touch and how you interpret touching, both in your personal and professional life.

2. Review Chapter 6 on client behaviors, especially in relation to approaching the client, since the behavior pattern may influence the client's response to touch.

3. Experiment with touch gradually if you are uncomfortable with it. For example, (a) extend your hand when meeting a new client, whether male or female; (b) use the "Indian" handshake, in which you place one hand in the client's hand and your other hand on top of the client's hand; (c) place your hand on the client's shoulder when speaking to him to provide touch in a physically neutral area; (d) touch the client lightly when asking him to awaken; and (e) if the client needs to have his cigarette lit, use this opportunity to touch by steadying his hand as you light his cigarette.

4. Become aware of how you touch and when you touch if you have been using touch in a mechanical fashion.

5. Develop a sense of your own body as you bathe, dress, or soothe an uncomfortable area. Since a great deal of personal touch is automatic, it takes effort to become consciously aware of when it occurs and your personal reaction to it.

6. Respect others' feelings about touch and learn to tell when someone is in a mood to be touched or to be left alone.

7. Remember that you have rights too, and that you can say "No" to someone else's desire to touch.

8. Discourage use of touch to cling. Suggest an appropriate alternative, such as a warm handshake.

9. Set limits on socially inappropriate touch by the client. Support touch that will be acceptable in the community.

10. Be aware of and respect cultural differences. Some cultures are very comfortable with touching; others are offended by touching with anyone other than their loved ones.

Touch is a way of staying in contact, a way of supporting reality, and a way of reducing loneliness. Basic care techniques, such as a back rub or foot massage, can go a long way in reaching or soothing a client. ". . . nonverbal communication should be encouraged since it is often the only pathway left to establish an interpersonal relationship with meaningful results" (Preston, 1973:2066).

USE OF HUMOR

One of the clearest definitions of humor is that offered by Joel Goodman (1981:4): "Humor is a set of attitudes and skills that we can use to move from 'grin and bear it' to 'grin and share it.'" It is an indirect form of communication, which, despite the mirth that is conveyed in the concept, is serious business. The effectiveness of the use of humor is related to timing, spontaneity, and the sender's intent.

According to Henn (1983:5), humor is a powerful tool that can serve as:

1. a tension releaser to avoid the build-up of stress. For example: In a busy psychiatric unit in a mental health center, a nurse commented, "As the Center Turns" parodying the soap opera, "As the World Turns." This was just enough to break the tension in the rather stressful situation. Laughter and tension are incompatible. Laughter causes the muscles to relax, and it is difficult to be anxious or tense when the muscles are limp. Also, research has revealed that laughter stimulates the brain to produce an arousal hormone, which in turn causes the release of endorphins, the body's natural painkillers (Peter and Dana, 1982:9).

2. an insight device that can help clients gain a new perspective on problems and explore other solutions. For example, by blowing up an event to the point of its being

ridiculous, an individual can sometimes see how irrational his thinking is. A child who breaks a lamp tells his mother that it broke because the table was in his way. The mother scolds the table for being in the way of the child; the child begins to laugh. He may think his mother is a little strange but he realizes, at the same time, how ridiculous his remark was and begins to assume responsibility for his behavior.

3.   an avenue of expression that can improve communication and relationships. For example, a client is obsessed with the idea that she "is burning up"; however, she has quite a collection of jokes. Her delusional system can be interrupted by asking her to tell a joke; as a result, communication is improved.

4.   a medium through which trust can be achieved, thus enhancing self-confidence and understanding. For example, a client who is mentally retarded uses a barrage of jokes in his relationships with staff, including the "knock-knock, who's there" sayings. Usually, staff respond by indicating that they don't know the answer. The client receives great pleasure in giving the correct response to his jokes. In this way, he experiences a bond with staff, along with self-confidence and security.

Norman Cousins, in his *Anatomy of an Illness as Perceived by the Patient* (1979:82, 84), relates the part that humor played in the lives of Dr. Albert Schweitzer and Sigmund Freud. It was customary for Dr. Schweitzer to present an amusing story at mealtime when staff came together as a way of reducing the effects of the temperatures, humidity, and tensions. Freud believed that humor was a useful way of dealing with nervous tension and could be used as an effective therapy.

How might the health provider use humor most effectively? Kaye Herth, in her article, "Laughter: A Nursing Rx" (1984:991), suggests doing an assessment of the client's receptivity to humor. She developed a humor history form that can be incorporated into the health history or filled out separately by the client. Some of the questions that can be included in such a form are: What part did humor play in the client's family as he was growing up? Was the client teased a lot as a child? What kind of joke does the client like? What makes him laugh? How often does he laugh? What is his favorite joke? After the form is filled out, the health provider should review it with the client and write a specific approach for laughter that is unique for that client. Other techniques that Herth used were:

1.   Having the client draw or visualize the present situation as a cartoon, exaggerating it so it is ridiculous. By injecting some humor into the situation, the client may be able to deal with it more effectively.

2.   Sharing with the client whatever brings him joy or laughter, such as a favorite book, record, picture, or story. The idea is to use these resources to get through the rough times.

Humor can be destructive and, if not used properly, can be a dangerous weapon. It is important to examine whose needs are being met with humor—the provider's or the client's? There is a humor referred to as gallows humor that is used when individuals or groups are faced with dangerous or very stressful situations, such as war, concentration camps, and life and death struggles. "Freud's basic concept that joking relieves repressed impulses and anxieties, and that laughter converts the unpleasant feelings to pleasant ones, underlies the theory of 'gallows humor'" (Robinson, 1977:61). Usually this humor is used to support one's own need and can be helpful as a coping technique. A good example of the use of gallows humor is in the well-known television series *M*A*S*H*. The staff's need for humor to survive difficult situations is demonstrated very clearly; however, the staff never puts down, depreciates, or laughs at any patient. Rarely is harm done by laughing *with* someone. It is when we laugh *at* someone that we exclude that person from the network of understanding and support. It is helpful for the health provider to assess his sense of humor: the situations in which it occurs, his frame of mind when it occurs, his emotional state at the time.

In the total plan of care for the client, "humor is *one* communication tool, *one* mechanism for coping. . . . It is useful and therapeutic in the right situation and the right time. . . . What is important is to understand humor, to become skilled in recognizing when it is appropriate and beneficial, and to encourage, not ignore, it" (Robinson, 187).

REFERENCES

Amacher, N.J., 1973. Touch is a way of caring. Am J Nurs, Vol. 75, No. 5, pp. 852–854.

Benson, H., 1976. The Relaxation Response. New York, Avon.

Berkowitz, L., 1973. The case for bottling up rage. Psychol Today, July, pp. 24–31.

Bolysenko, J., 1984. Ways to control stress and make it work for you. U.S. News World Rep, pp. 69–70.

Burnside, I.M., 1973. Touching is talking. Am J Nurs, Vol. 73, No. 12, pp. 2060–2063.

Clark, C., 1981. Inner dialogue: A self-healing approach for nurses and clients. Am J Nurs, Vol. 81, No. 6, pp. 1191–1193.

Cousins, N., 1979. Anatomy of an Illness as Perceived by the Patient. New York, W.W. Norton and Co.

Davis, M., McKay, M., and Eshelman E., 1981. The Relaxation and Stress Reduction Workbook. Richmond, Calif., New Harbinger Publications.

DeThomaso, M.T., 1971. Touch power and the screen of loneliness. Perspect Psychiatr Care, Vol. 9, No. 3, pp. 112–118.

DiMotto, J., 1984. Relaxation. Am J Nurs, Vol. 84, No. 6, pp. 754–758.

Donnelly, G., 1980. Relax? That's easy for you to say! RN, June, pp. 34–80.

Donnelly, G., 1980. Progressive relaxation? But, that sounds like work. RN, August, pp. 34–36.

Flaherty, G., and Fitzpatrick, J., 1978. Relaxation techniques to increase comfort level of postoperative patients: A preliminary study. Nurs Res, November/December, Vol. 27, No. 6, pp. 352–355.

Gagan, J., 1984. Imagery: An overview with suggested application for nursing. Perspect Psychiatr Care, Vol. 22, No. 1, pp. 20–22.

Goodman, J., 1981. Laughing Matters, Vol. 1, No. 1, pp. 1–39. Saratoga Springs, N.Y., The Humor Project.

Henn, M.B., 1983. Intervening with humor. Free Assoc, Vol. 10, No. 2, March/April.

Herth, K., 1984. Laughter: A nursing Rx. Am J Nurs, Vol. 84, No. 8, pp. 991–992.

Huss, J., 1977. 1976. Eleanor Clark Slagle Lecture: Touch with caring or a caring touch? Am J Occup Ther, Vol. 31, No. 1, pp. 11–18.

Hutchinson, S.A., 1976. Humor: A link to life. In Kneisl, C.R. (ed.): Current Perspectives in Psychiatric Nursing: Issues and Trends. St. Louis, C.V. Mosby, pp. 201–210.

Jacobson, E., 1964. Anxiety and Tension Control. Philadelphia, J.B. Lippincott.

Lazarus, A., 1977. In the Mind's Eye. New York, Rawson Associates.

Leuner, H., 1969. Guided affective imagery. Am J Psychother, Vol. 23, No. 1, pp. 4–22.

McGough, E., 1974. The silent language that reveals all: Touch. Fam Circle, August, pp. 2, 4, 48 and 124.

Moody, R. Jr., 1978. Laugh After Laugh, The Healing Power of Humor. Philadelphia, J.B. Lippincott.

Osterlund, H., 1983. Humor: A serious approach to patient care. Nursing 83, December, pp. 46–47.

Peter, L., and Dana, B., 1982. The Laughter Prescription: The Tools of Humor and How to Use Them. New York, Ballantine Books.

Preston, T., 1973. When words fail. Am J Nurs, Vol. 73, No. 12, pp. 2064–2066.

Risberg, G., 1984. The Importance of Touching. Seminar, Green Bay, WI.

Robinson, V., 1977. Humor and the Health Professions. Thorofare, N.J., Charles B. Slack.

Roon, K., 1961. Karin Roon's New Way to Relax. New York, Greystone Press.

Schiralde, G., 1982. Facts to Relax By. Provo, Utah, Utah Valley Hospital.

Selye, H., 1965. The stress syndrome. Am J Nurs, Vol. 65, No. 3, pp. 97–99.

Simonton, C., Simonton, S., and Creighton, J., 1978. Getting Well Again. Los Angeles, J.P. Tarcher.

Trygstad, L., 1980. Simple ways to help anxious patients, RN, December, pp. 28–32.

Tuttle, K., 1982. Facts to Relax By. Schiralde C. (ed.), Provo, Utah, Utah Valley Hospital, p. 81.

Vissing, Y., and Burke M., 1984. Visualization techniques for health care workers. J Psychosoc Nurs Ment Health Serv, January, Vol. 22, No. 1, January, pp. 29–32.

Warner, S., 1984. Humor and self-disclosure within the milieu. J Psychosoc Nurs, Vol. 22, No. 4, pp. 17–21.

17

PHYSICAL CARE AND NUTRITION

LEARNING OBJECTIVES—Upon completing this chapter, the reader will be able to:

1. Explain the physical care required for clients with specific patterns of behavior.

2. Describe the relationship of nutrition to mental health.

PHYSICAL CARE

The client's physical care is threefold: (1) maintain reasonable health, (2) maintain physical safety, and (3) maintain social acceptability. The health provider's function will vary depending on the client's mental and physical condition. At different times it will include providing complete care, teaching the client how to do his own care, and, finally, occasionally reminding the client about the need for physical care. The client's admission assessment must include an evaluation of the client's nutrition, elimination, sleep and rest, grooming, and special problems.

The health provider's attitude in assisting or teaching the client about his physical care sets the stage for client compliance. The client, no matter how psychotic, quickly senses whether the health provider is a respectful advocate who will assist with his care until he is able to care for himself again.

Table 17–1 emphasizes the significant aspects of physical care for persons with problem behaviors.

TABLE 17–1. Problems in Physical Care for Clients with Specific Patterns of Behavior

PHYSICAL CARE	ANXIOUS PATTERN OF BEHAVIOR
Nutrition	Vomiting, fear of dishes or food, lengthy rituals may prevent adequate intake of food and fluids. Advance reminding of mealtime will provide time to complete lengthy rituals.
Elimination	Check daily weight and intake and output on client who is vomiting. Poor nutritional intake may affect elimination; monitor initially.
Sleep and Rest	High anxiety, extensive rituals, somatic concerns may prevent adequate sleep and rest. Client needs advance reminder to complete rituals prior to bedtime. Use relaxation at bedtime.
Grooming	May require total physical care and reminders at times. Paralysis may interfere with ability to do care. Frequently diaphoretic; check for skin breakdown.
Special Problems	Rule out real physical problem without feeding the pathology. Check out physical problems when client is not complaining.
PHYSICAL CARE	**DEPRESSED PATTERN OF BEHAVIOR**
Nutrition	May not eat or drink because of lack of appetite; feels undeserving or has somatic delusions regarding physical problems that he thinks make eating impossible. Sit with client; encourage and/or feed at first. Needs small meals with dietary supplements and fluids.

TABLE 17-1. Problems in Physical Care for Clients with Specific Patterns of Behavior—*Continued*

Elimination	May forget to void. Check for distended bladder. Take to bathroom regularly; remind to void. Check for constipation. Monitor toileting. Increase water, juices, fruit, and activity.
Sleep and Rest	Disturbed, unsatisfying sleep. May sleep too little or too much. Provide for a short nap daily, but discourage long periods of bed rest during the day. A backrub at bedtime is relaxing and provides touch as well.
Grooming	Neglects appearance. Needs help with bathing, shampooing, setting hair, shaving, oral hygiene, nail care, foot care. Skin may be in poor condition due to poor food and fluid intake. Check initially.
Special Problems	Dehydration always is a concern with severe depression. Check for poor skin turgor, dry skin, scanty urine, thickened secretions. Check results of blood work and urinalysis. Immediate medical intervention may be needed.
PHYSICAL CARE	**AGGRESSIVE (MANIC) PATTERN OF BEHAVIOR**
Nutrition	Too busy to eat or drink. May throw food. As likely to starve as a client who is depressed. Seat away from others. Serve finger foods that can be eaten on the run. Offer high-calorie liquids initially.
Elimination	Monitor elimination; may be too "busy" to toilet self.
Sleep and Rest	Lack of sleep is a serious problem. Continuous activity may result in death due to fatigue, coronary insufficiency, and other related causes (Payne and Clunn, 1977: 83). Needs extra rest periods: soothing warm baths, quiet music, nonstimulating colors, and someone sitting with him on a 1:1 basis may promote rest.
Grooming	Needs a great deal of help. Too busy to groom self. Perspires profusely due to frantic activity. May experience skin breakdown. Frequently has minor cuts and bruises. Tends to "decorate" self. Uses too much make-up. Needs suggestions on more acceptable hygienic practices and clothing.
Special Problems	Needs to be checked and monitored physically when acutely ill: blood work, urinalysis, vital signs, intake, and output.
PHYSICAL CARE	**WITHDRAWAL PATTERN OF BEHAVIOR (AS OBSERVED IN SCHIZOPHRENIA)**
Nutrition	May not eat or drink because of lack of interest. Severe regression resulting in inability to eat or fear of eating. May need to be fed initially. Offer small amounts of fluids frequently between meals.
Elimination	May retain feces and urine. Needs regular reminding and monitoring.
Sleep and Rest	Frequently disturbed; has difficulty sleeping or staying awake. Evaluate reason individually. For example, going to bed during the day may be a form of withdrawal that needs to be interrupted to support reality.
Grooming	Frequently will not initiate personal care. Responds to step-by-step directions on doing care. Check skin carefully, since client may be unaware of injuries when very withdrawn. Difficulty making clothing choices; offer choice of two items.
Special Problems	Lack of personal care may result in physical problems. Follow through on checking out abnormal physical signs. Decreased perception of pain stimuli, such as hot and cold, may lead to injuries. Needs additional supervision in bathing and smoking.
PHYSICAL CARE	**OVERLY SUSPICIOUS PATTERN OF BEHAVIOR**
Nutrition	May not eat for fear of being poisoned. Let him prepare his own meal or serve himself, or serve food in closed containers. Offer to taste food with utensil of his choice if he requests.
Elimination	Usually not a problem unless related to lack of food and fluids due to delusions.
Sleep and Rest	Disturbed because of fear of sleeping or fear of sleeping in room with others. Have him sleep alone; if this doesn't work, consider hallway. As one client remarked, "No one will dare hurt me with so many people around!"
Grooming	Usually not a problem. May be suspicious of health provider's attempt to help. Offer, but do not encourage vigorously. Will be more receptive when delusional pattern begins to subside.
Special Problems	Tends to identify himself as a staff person rather than as a client. Therefore, implementing any physical care is a challenge.

NUTRITION*

The objectives of nutritional care for the hospitalized client are threefold: (1) prevention or correction of malnutrition, (2) correction of feeding problems, and (3) restoration of the client's ability to eat with emotional satisfaction (Zeman, 1983:611). To support these objectives, the health provider must understand some basic facts about nutrients and, more specifically, about nutrition and emotional stress.

Nutrition can be described as a science that investigates food, including aspects such as the physiological and psychological reasons for choosing certain foods we eat, causes of overeating and undereating, and the evaluation of diets for adequate nutrient density. Nutrition also studies the exact function of the individual nutrients obtained from food inside the body.

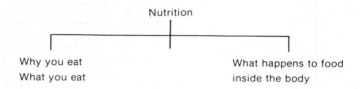

There are six basic classifications of nutrients, each with its own function within the body. Table 17–2 identifies each nutrient and explains briefly the nutrient's function.

TABLE 17–2. Nutrients and their Functions

NUTRIENT	FUNCTION
Carbohydrates	Provide heat and energy. Protein-sparing. Assist in fat metabolism.
Proteins	Build and repair tissue (only nutrient with this function). Assist body in resisting diseases. Provide heat and energy. Contribute to body secretions and fluids.
Fats	Concentrated source of heat and energy. Carry fat-soluble vitamins A, D, E, and K. Aid in normal tissue functioning. Provide feelings of satiety in diet. Reserve fuel supply. Maintain body temperature by insulating. Hold organs in place and prevent injury.
Vitamins	Promote growth. Aid in producing healthy tissue. Resist infections. Aid in vital body processes.
Minerals	Necessary part of all cells and body fluids. Form structural framework of body as part of bones and teeth. Assist in acid-base balance and osmotic pressure. Regulate metabolism of enzymes. Assist in nerve impulse transmission.
Water	Solvent that aids in softening and liquifying foods. Regulates body temperature. Transports nutrients and body secretions throughout the body. Excretory agent adds bulk to intestinal tract. Lubricant: moves parts of body surrounded with water to prevent friction and wear (Adapted from Williams, 1984).

It is known that these nutrients affect not only physical health but intellectual functioning as well. For example, several nutrients are highly involved in the functioning of the central nervous system. Severe protein deficiency during pregnancy can lead to mental retardation in the infant. Cretinism, characterized by severe mental retardation, is known to be related to severe iodine deficiency during pregnancy. Nutritional deficiencies during infancy and early childhood are related to learning disabilities. Protein-calorie malnutrition may lead to mental retardation. While these relationships are clear-cut and based on scientific study, the relationship between nutritional deficiency and mental illness is not as well-defined. It is generally accepted that well-nourished individuals are better

*This section was written with the assistance of Terri Timmers, R.D.

able to cope with stress than those who are poorly nourished. Whether this applies to all forms of stress is unknown at this time. Kipp (1984:1) states that "If an individual is marginally deficient in a nutrient, the stress may exacerbate the condition. Undernutrition is in itself a stress, and the body undergoes adaptation to maintain equilibrium and adequate functional status when only a limited supply of nutrients is available. When additional stress is then superimposed on the already adapted state, the individual no longer has the same reserve capacity to adapt to the stress." Some of the symptoms of nutritional deficiency are similar to symptoms of mental illness. Table 17–3 lists these symptoms.

TABLE 17-3. Symptoms of Nutritional Deficiency

NUTRIENT	SYMPTOMS OF DEFICIENCY
Thiamine (vitamin B_1)	Irritability, inability to concentrate, lack of appetite, depression, fatigue, hysteria, uncoordinated gait.
Niacin	Loss of appetite, lack of energy, irritability, confusion, delusions, hallucination
Pantothenic acid	Depression
Pyridoxine (vitamin B_6)	Hyperirritability, depression, sullenness
Folic acid	Irritability, forgetfulness
Cobalamin (vitamin B_{12})	Depression, mental deterioration (Robinson, 1983)

This is not to imply that nutritional deficiencies cause mental illness. Furthermore, "evidence to indicate an increased need for nutrients during stress is not well established" (Kipp, 1984: 2). The Recommended Dietary Allowance (RDA) levels of nutrients are, at this time, considered to adequately meet the daily nutritional requirements and continue to be the basis for determining a balanced diet for the client. However, the health provider must remember that the client's nutritional state and eating habits must be assessed at the time of admission and attended to with the help of the dietary department.

Eating habits leading to overnutrition or undernutrition may have changed for a number of reasons. Table 17–4 indicates briefly some of these changes and possible nutritional interventions.

ALCOHOL AND NUTRITION

Alcohol is high in calories, but it has no food value. Alcohol provides 7 to 10 percent of total calories in an average American's diet. It may even provide a much larger percentage of calories in the diet long before a person is considered alcoholic. A male consuming 2500 calories per day and drinking four or five beers a day would be receiving about 25 percent of his calories from alcohol. This is not a totally uncommon practice. Alcoholics frequently drink instead of eating a balanced diet. Alcohol can also increase excretion of nutrients and decrease their use in the body. This, in turn, leads to decreased levels of nutrients in body tissues. Abnormalities will develop if the level of nutrients are not in the proper concentration for adequate tissue function. Malnutritional diseases may result. Alcohol is an irritant to all cells of the body. Consequently, all systems of the body are affected in some way. Only the systems directly affected nutritionally will be discussed in this segment.

After one takes a drink, alcohol is absorbed almost completely into the bloodstream. The body identifies it as a toxin that must be removed from the bloodstream. Most of it (i.e., 70 to 90 percent) is metabolized in the liver. The products of alcohol breakdown can interfere with normal function of the liver. This can cause problems with bile formation, storage of vitamins and minerals, and proper use of proteins and fats. Fatty liver can result from the liver's inability to utilize fats. Chronic alcohol consumption along with

TABLE 17-4. Patterns of Behavior and Nutritional Interventions

CLIENT PATTERN OF BEHAVIOR	POTENTIAL PROBLEM	NUTRITIONAL INTERVENTION
Alcohol Dependent	Avitamosis: May be malnourished (even though weight may not show it). May experience dehydration due to the diuretic affect of alcohol.	Additional vitamin B_6, B_{12}, thiamine, folic acid, niacin initially ordered by physician. May benefit from class on nutrition and alcohol consumption. Needs additional liquids—fruit juice especially good. Responds to eating with peers after detoxification is complete.
Anxious	May overeat or undereat or may have developed rigid eating pattern. Faces problem of overnutrition or undernutrition.	Limit calories, or, if undereating, offer one food with one utensil at a time if client is having difficulty deciding what to eat. Sit with him. May need food supplements initially and frequent small meals throughout day.
Depressed (Suicidal)	May overeat initially or undereat when severely depressed because he feels he does not deserve to eat or because of somatic delusions of not being able to eat or of being very ill. Faces problem of undernutrition and dehydration.	Sit with client. Small servings do not seem as overwhelming. May use paper plates and plastic utensils initially; take utensils away when finished. May need to feed client initially or add food supplement until regular eating resumes.
Overactive (Manic)	Lack of time to eat or drink. Faces problem of undernutrition and dehydration.	Isolate client from others. Sit with him. If unable to sit still, walk with him. Offer finger foods and sips of fluid frequently throughout the day.
Overly Suspicious	Concern that food may be poisoned. Faces problem of undernutrition and dehydration.	Provide choices of foods; allow client to serve himself; use closed containers or taste food if requested by client.
Behavior Related to Organic Brain Changes	May be confused or forgetful. Faces problem of undernutrition and dehydration.	Sit with client. Offer direction. Feed if necessary. Use small spoonfuls. Offer liquids in between. Allow adequate chewing time: decreased saliva due to medication may hamper chewing and swallowing.
Withdrawal Pattern (as seen in schizophrenia)	May experience delusions regarding food or lack interest in eating. Check for dehydration and weight loss.	May initially do better eating by self. Direct or fill one spoonful at a time if needed. May need planned dietary supplements and snacks until eating normally.
Mentally Retarded with Emotional Disturbance	Depending on level of functioning, may stuff mouth with food; risk of choking; overeating may lead to vomiting. Steals food from others' plates.	May have to offer one food with one utensil at a time. Teach to place one hand on the lap while eating with the other. Sit with him. Offer positive verbal reinforcement. Add one food at a time until client can deal with whole meal. (This is a slow process; program must be followed faithfully in order to succeed.)

malnutrition may cause toxic liver damage (cirrhosis). Alcohol stimulates the pancreas to make pancreatic juice and enzymes but blocks passage of this juice into the small intestine. Chronic alcohol use can cause enzymes to digest the pancreas. The pancreas also produces insulin; lack of enzymes and insulin can cause severe malnutrition and diabetes. Other chronic nutritional affects of alcohol include decreased ability of the blood to clot due to lack of vitamin K and brittle bones due to lack of calcium. Korsakoff's disease, also known as alcohol amnestic disorder, is caused by thiamine deficiency associated with prolonged heavy alcohol use. It is characterized by memory loss and thought disorder and often follows an acute episode of Wernicke's encephalopathy. Wernicke's disease is a neurologic disease manifested by confusion, ataxia, eye movement abnormalities, and other neurologic symptoms. If Wernicke's disease is treated early with large doses of thiamine, alcohol amnestic disorder may not develop (APA, 1980:136–137).

Because of the diuretic effect of alcohol, adequate hydration is important when dealing with the alcoholic client. Each facility has its own protocol for dealing with hydration.

EATING DISORDERS

A special type of nutritional problem is presented by the client with eating disorders. This group of disorders includes anorexia nervosa, bulimia, and bulimarexia. The disorders are characterized by gross disturbances in eating behavior. In anorexia nervosa, self-imposed starvation leads to emaciation, nutritional deficiency disorder, and atrophic changes. "The essential features are intense fears of becoming obese, disturbances of body image, significant weight loss, refusal to maintain a minimum body weight and amenorrhea (in females). The disturbance cannot be accounted for by a known physical disorder" (APA, 1980:67). All of the individuals, usually teen-age females, perceive themselves as being fat, regardless of their weight. A 25 percent loss of the original body weight is an important factor in diagnosis. This is often accomplished by reduced food intake, especially of high carbohydrate and high fat foods; self-induced vomiting; use of laxatives or diuretics; and extensive exercising. Individuals who are unable to continuously maintain the low caloric intake often go on eating binges followed by self-induced vomiting. Hospitalization is often necessary to prevent starvation.

Bulimia is characterized by "episodic binge eating accompanied by an awareness that the eating pattern is abnormal, fear of not being able to stop eating voluntarily, and depressed mood- and self-deprecating thoughts following the eating binges" (APA, 1980: 67). Clients with bulimia usually are very concerned about their weight and control it through dieting, vomiting, cathartics, or diuretics. Complications associated with bulimia include dehydration, malnutrition, electrolyte imbalance, and dental enamel erosion.

Bulimarexia is a starvation-purge syndrome. The client may be of normal or near normal weight. In some clients, it follows an episode of anorexia. Other clients may develop bulimarexia after a diet. Physical symptoms, such as abdominal bloating, excess gas, and acne, may result from mineral deficiency. The gastric acid irritates tissue and dissolves teeth.

The dietitian's role in nutritional assessment and rehabilitation is an important part of the team effort in dealing with the client with eating disorders. It requires patience, the development of a trusting relationship, and knowledge that the regimen must be instituted slowly to allow the client's body to adjust to the increased intake. The client with anorexia frequently has an above-average understanding of nutrition but does not connect information about nutritional requirements with her own body. "They have difficulty relating to physical and emotional feelings, so they often deny feelings of hunger, discomfort or fatigue" (MPI, 1984: 4). The client with bulimia needs "reassurance that the return to normal eating means weight maintenance, not weight gain" (MPI, 1984:4).

REFERENCES

Diagnostic and Statistical Manual of Mental Disorders–III. Washington, American Psychiatric Association, 1980.

Kipp, D., 1984. Stress and nutrition. Contemp Nutr, July, Vol. 9, No. 7.

Anorexia nervosa: The relentless pursuit of thinness. Milwaukee Psychiatric Hospital, Prog Notes, Winter, 1984, Vol. 1, Issue 3.

Payne, D., and Clunn, P., 1977. Psychiatric Mental Health Nursing: Nursing Outline Series. 2nd ed. Garden City, N.Y., Medical Examination.

Williams, S.R., 1984. Mowry's Basic Nutrition & Diet Therapy. 7th ed. St. Louis, Times Mirror/Mosby College Publishing.

Zeman, F.J., 1983. Clinical Nutrition and Dietetics. Lexington, Mass., Collamore Press.

18

GUIDELINES FOR DEALING WITH THE PHYSICALLY ASSAULTIVE PERSON

LEARNING OBJECTIVES—Upon completing this chapter, the reader will be able to:

1. Give six guidelines for dealing with the physically assaultive person.

Much of the effective handling of the physically assaultive person is related to the mental attitude of the health provider who is caring for that person. Therefore, there will be considerable emphasis on the health provider's knowledge of self in relation to physical limitations and emotional weaknesses, events that would cause the provider to become emotionally upset. "Whenever emotional upset occurs, the brain shuts off" (Gorski and Miller, 1981:4). If there are emotional weaknesses, it is important for the provider to learn to desensitize reactions to these areas. Through this self-understanding, the understanding of the client's behavior, and the understanding that assaultiveness is a response to real or perceived situations, many potentially assaultive situations can be prevented.

The guidelines for dealing with physically assaultive persons are from a study on critical behaviors conducted by the American Institutes for Research (Jacobs, Gamel, and Brotz, 1973:16).

1. The health provider should intervene immediately when the client needs controls or limits. This may mean just separating the client from what seems to be irritating him. If intervention is not immediate, the client's behavior will continue to escalate until his emotions take over and he loses control.

2. Approach the client in a nonthreatening manner; allow him physical space. Each individual has his own personal space, which is sometimes referred to as one's "bubble." When someone is emotionally disturbed, this bubble enlarges and becomes a protective device; to trespass into this area is very threatening to the individual. Here, the health provider's posture is significant: avoid hands on hips, clenched fists, and hands folded across the chest in an authoritarian manner.

3. Refrain from reacting solely on an emotional basis. If the health provider responds emotionally, then the client becomes lost because the provider is busy taking care of his own needs. The client is very perceptive of the provider's weak spots because of his sensitivity and past experiences. When a client becomes disturbed, he attacks these weak areas. The behavior is similar to a child who acts out when his mother is not feeling well and is most vulnerable.

4. Be firm but understanding; do not show fear. Fear is a highly significant factor, since the client who is emotionally distraught usually strikes out to protect himself. If the health provider is frightened, then the client feels insecure and will

become more aggressive to protect himself because he cannot depend on the provider for his protection. The health provider should use a calm, but firm, manner in approaching the client and attempting to talk him down. Comments can be made such as, "It seems that you are really upset about something," or "Let's sit down and talk about what's bothering you. How about a glass of juice?" In this way, the health provider offers the client an alternative to his assaultive behavior.

5. Consistently enforce limits. It is important for the provider to communicate to the client that he will not allow the client to hurt himself or others. Statements such as, "I cannot allow you to injure yourself, other clients, or me," or "I know that you don't want to hit me," let the client know that the health provider will protect him. These statements must be made in a sincere, calm, and secure tone of voice in order to be effective.

6. Refrain from arguing with or further provoking the client. These interactions only cause the client's behavior to escalate and further complicate the situation. Once the emotions take over, a rational approach becomes impossible.

7. Attempt to discover the cause for the client's disturbance. Rather than a distortion of what the client is perceiving, the reason for the client's assaultiveness might have a very legitimate basis. Some of these reasons could be failure to receive a promised visit from a relative, fear of another client, inconsistent and conflicting approaches to the client, health providers' behavior that is disturbing to the client, a lack of trust in the health provider, and a reaction to psychotropic medication.

8. Help the client verbalize his feelings and discuss his problems. The health provider needs to provide the setting and opportunity for the client to talk about what is bothering him and to explore other options that might be helpful in working through his problems.

9. Remove the client to a nonstimulating, safe environment. Environment has a great influence on behavior. Flashing lights and loud music can excite individuals, while dim lights, soft music, and subdued colors can be very relaxing. One of the best places to take a client is probably to his room or to a small sitting room that is removed from the main center of activity.

10. Reassure, support, calm, and soothe the client. Communicate to him that he will not be allowed to lose control and that his behavior can be contained. If appropriate, some comment relating to the cause of the disturbance might be made, such as, "It must be upsetting not to have your family visit you," or "It must be confusing and upsetting to you not to be able to go home this weekend when you were able to go home last weekend."

11. Provide appropriate diversion. Because the client who is emotionally disturbed has a short attention span, diversion can be a helpful technique in working with an assaultive client. Examples of diversions include involving the client in playing cards, watching television, taking a walk, doing an art or craft project, and helping the health provider with a necessary task. Or the health provider can offer the client some nourishment or a cigarette if he smokes, or just talk to him about some interest of his (e.g., sports, cars, books). Physical diversion techniques, such as throwing a towel, sheet, or coat over the client's head, may be necessary if the client becomes physically assaultive.

12. Provide the client with physical activity. One of the best outlets for excess energy is strenuous physical activity. Activities such as hitting a punching bag, swimming, shooting baskets, and playing ping pong provide a means for the client to express negative feelings constructively.

13. Through actions, assure the client that his behavior has not alienated the health provider. The health provider must communicate to the client that he *is accepted as an individual* but that the health provider does not approve of the client's behavior. This is an important distinction for the health provider to make because the client usually operates from the premise that the health provider doesn't like his behavior and, therefore, doesn't like him.

14. Encourage the client to understand, control, and accept responsibility for his behavior. If the health provider treats the client as though he expects the client to be in control of himself, the client is more likely to be so. Remind the client of the consequences of unacceptable behavior. Also let the client know that he makes the decision about his behavior and, as a result, is responsible for decisions.

15. Reinforce positive behavior. Focusing on the client's strengths increases his self-esteem, establishes trust, and makes him feel more secure. Many times the client is unaware of his positive qualities because so much emphasis is placed on the negative aspects of his behavior. Use positive reinforcement whenever possible. For example, point out to the client that he made a good decision or selected a nice shirt to wear. The continuous use of positive reinforcement should decrease the client's need to be assaultive. For examples of client/provider interactions, refer to Physical and Verbal Aggressiveness in the Index of Specific Behaviors, Chapter 5.

When it is necessary to intervene physically when a client is assaultive, the health provider must remember that for anything to be accomplished physically, it must first be accomplished mentally. The health provider mentally rehearses the successful outcome of his intervention. This is important because if the provider does not visualize successful management of the situation, it will not become a reality. Every situation is different. However, some basic points should be remembered whenever a health provider intervenes with a physically assaultive client.

1. Defensive techniques are learned and therefore must be practiced until they become part of the provider's automatic reaction to assault. This is particularly important, since sometimes during physical assault things happen quickly.

2. Don't try to be a hero. Get out of the way and get help, if possible.

3. The health provider should place one foot forward and angle the rear foot to the outside. This provides a firm base of support to help the provider maintain his balance if pushed.

4. Keep a proper distance from the client. Maintain eye contact and relaxed posture with arms loose. All these factors are less threatening to a client. Also, if in a room, the provider should not stand in a corner without a ready exit. At the same time, the client should be able to exit and not feel cornered, since this can be very threatening.

5. Always work against the weakest point of any hold, using arms as levers.

6. Use arms and hands to protect the face and head, turn the thigh sideways to protect the groin area.

Some general physical interventions will be described. However, to be effective, these defensive techniques must be practiced under *qualified supervision*. No technique is a guarantee that injury will be avoided.

1. The wrist grab. The weak point of a wrist grab is between the client's thumb and fingers. The wrist can be removed by moving it against the thumb of the attacker's hand. Sometimes a client grabs a wrist for support or to be close to someone. Before implementing the wrist release, evaluate the situation. After a

short time, the client may let go. If he doesn't, and the grip is bothersome, kindly ask the client to release his grip before implementing the technique.

2. Clothing grab. If a client grabs clothing, place one hand under and close to the grasping hand to keep the clothing against the body. With the other hand, push the client's grasping wrist off in the direction of its knuckles. This technique will protect clothing from being torn.

3. Hair grabs. When hair is grabbed, it is important to prevent pulling of the hair. This can best be done by interlocking the fingers over the attacker's hands and pressing down with the palms of the hands. This will alleviate the pain from the grabbing of the hair. This technique needs to be demonstrated for actual release of the attacker's fingers, since it involves bending the body down and around, depending on whether the hair is grabbed from the front or rear. However, a co-worker can use the assist (see below), which is helpful in getting the attacker to release his fingers.

4. The assist (Foster, 1979: Workshop). The assist involves coming up behind the attacker and placing one hand over the attacker's eyes. The other hand pulls the attacker backwards and down, using the thigh to guide the attacker to the floor. The attacker, in an effort to regain his balance and vision, will usually release his hands.

5. Chokes. The most important thing to remember in a choke is to keep the airway open. Keeping the chin down will help relieve pressure on the trachea. If choked from the front, make a fist with both hands. Then, with considerable force, bring the clasped hands up through the attacker's forearms. This will usually release the attacker's grip. It is important, then, to step back and away from the client.

6. Human bites. Human bites are very dangerous. Because of the bacteria in the human mouth, broken skin should be treated immediately to prevent infection. Again, as in the hair grab, do not pull away; instead, move into the attacker's mouth. Release can usually be obtained by gently pressing the forefinger into the attacker's cheek until the finger can be felt between the attacker's teeth. The assist can be used to encourage the attacker to release his bite.

7. Escorting clients.
    a. For a mildly excited client, the provider can walk beside the client, using his outside arm to hold the client's wrist that is next to the provider's body. The provider's other arm, which is next to the client, is placed around the client's waist, grasping the other forearm. In this way, the provider can gently guide the client (Fig. 18–1).
    b. To control an excited client when alone, the provider can grab both of the client's wrists from behind and pull his arms around him. It is important for the provider's left hand to grasp the client's right wrist, and vice versa. The client's left arm should be below his right arm so he cannot move his arm back and forth. This is called the basket hold (Figure 18–2). If the person is taller than the provider, more control can be obtained if the center of gravity is lowered. This is done as the provider moves his knees into the back of the client's knees. In this way, the client can be lowered to the floor very gently (Fig. 18–3).
    c. If two providers are working with the client, one provider should stand on either side of the client. The provider's outside arm is brought across the

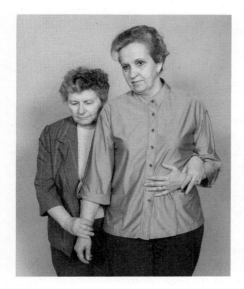

Figure 18-1. One-person escort for mild excitement.

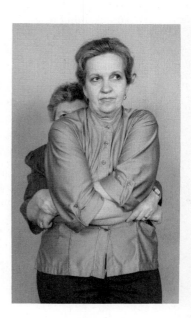

Figure 18-2. The basket hold.

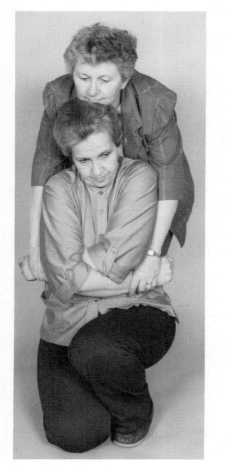

Figure 18-3. Lowering the center of gravity in the basket hold.

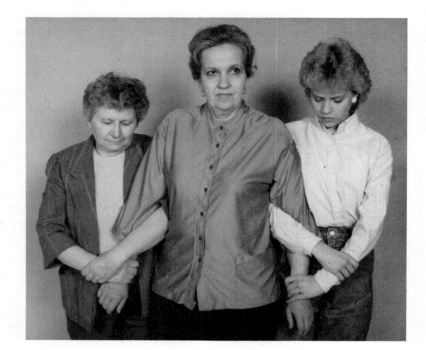

Figure 18-4. Two-person forward escort.

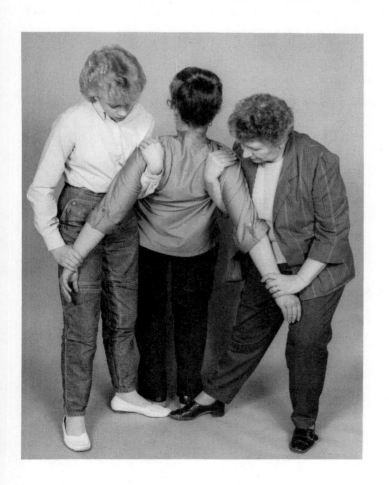

Figure 18-5. Two-person escort walking client backwards and lowering the center of gravity.

provider's body and clasps the client's wrist. The provider's other arm, which is next to the client, is brought between the client's arm and chest, clasping the wrist of the provider's outside arm. Staying close to the client's body decreases client movement (Fig. 18–4).

d. If a client is disturbed, it may be easier to walk him backwards. With the client facing backward and the two health providers facing forward, the providers hold the client's wrists with their outer hands. The providers' inner hands are brought up under the client's armpits, supporting his shoulders. Both providers use their feet to push the client's feet out, lowering the client's center of gravity. In this way, the client can be pulled backward without discomfort (Fig. 18–5).

Again, a word of caution is necessary. Reading about physical management techniques alone is not enough. They must be demonstrated and practiced. It is hoped that by following the suggested guidelines, assaultiveness will be avoided, and physical intervention will be unnecessary.

REFERENCES

Anders, R.L., 1977. When a patient becomes violent. Am J Nurs, Vol. 77, No. 7, pp. 1144–1148.

Barash, D.A., 1984. Defusing the violent patient—before he explodes. RN, March, pp. 34–37.

Barile, L., 1982. A model for teaching management of disturbed behavior. J Psychosoc Nurs Ment Health Serv, Vol. 20, No. 11, pp. 9–11.

Foster, R., 1979. Gentle Self Defense. Lawrence, KS, Camelot Behavioral Systems Workshop.

Gertz, B., 1980. Training for prevention of assaultive behavior in a psychiatric setting. Hosp Community Psychiatry, Vol. 31, No. 9, pp. 628–630.

Gorski, T., and Miller, M., 1981. The Management of Aggression and Violence. Hazel Crest, IL, Human Ecology Systems, Inc.

Jacobs, A.M., Gamel, N.M., and Bratz, C.A., 1973. Critical Behaviors in Psychiatric Mental Health Nursing. Palo Alto, CA, American Institute for Research, p. 16.

Karshmer, J., 1978. The application of social learning theory to aggression. Perspect Psychiatr Care, Vol. 16, Nos. 5–6, pp. 223–227.

Lathrop, V., 1978. Aggression as a response. Perspect Psychiatr Care, Vol. 16, Nos. 5–6, pp. 202–205.

Pisarcik, G., 1981. Facing the violent patient. Nursing 81, September, pp. 62–65.

Pribula, I., 1983. Disarming the agitated combative or destructive patient. Free Assoc. May/June, Vol. 10, No. 3, pp. 5–6.

Stewart, A., 1978. Handling the aggressive patient. Perspect Psychiatr Care, Vol. 16, Nos. 5–6, pp. 228–232.

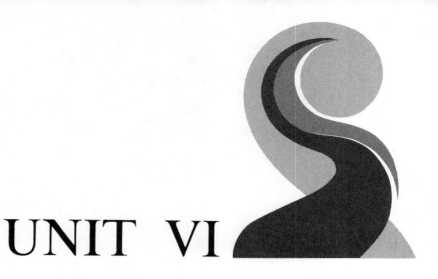

UNIT VI

EVALUATION EXERCISES

This part of the book is intended to assist the health provider in applying the material. Four varied exercises are offered to meet the provider's learning style.

Exercise 1 includes illustrations of behavior that represent behaviors described in the book. For each behavior, the provider is asked to state (1) his immediate feeling response to the situation and (2) his verbal and nonverbal response to the client. Criteria for evaluating the responses in this exercise focus on the understanding of behavior, as described below:

    1. The responses indicate the use of positive approaches suggested in the book.

    2. The responses do not support the client's pathological behavior.

Guidelines with some possible answers to the illustrated behaviors can be found at the end of the exercise. This exercise can be used as a pre- and/or post-evaluation tool.

Exercise 2 is the problem-solving process. Using the outline provided, the health provider is to take a problem and work it through. An example of how this is done appears in Chapter 2.

Exercise 3 is a positive approach to making the health provider aware of his behavior and of how it influences others' behavior. Any number of "Health Providers' Interactions That Enhance the Client's Human Dignity and Worth" can be selected.

In the sample of this exercise, five behaviors are listed with an opportunity for the health provider to score himself.

Exercise 4 is a crossword puzzle that covers certain aspects of material presented in the book.

EVALUATION EXERCISE 1

Situation A. Miss Eldridge is a 30-year-old woman with many physical complaints. All of her laboratory tests have been negative. She continuously paces back and forth. As she meets you in the hallway, she relates the following:

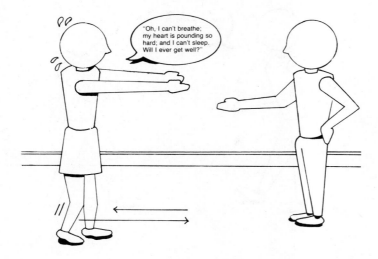

1. Give your immediate feeling response to the above situation.
2. Give your verbal and nonverbal response to the above situation.

Situation B. Mrs. Cannon is a 28-year-old woman who sits on the floor in the corner of the room and seldom speaks to anyone. Periodically, she will turn her head as if listening to someone and then speaks although no one is present. You are approaching her to take care of her needs.

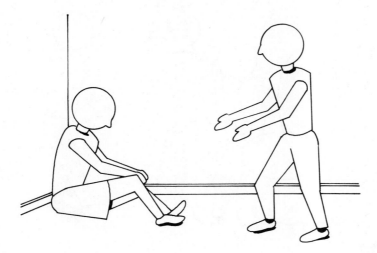

1. Give your immediate feeling response to the above situation.
2. Give your verbal and nonverbal response to the above situation.

Situation C. Mr. Heckel is a 19-year-old man who is very argumentative. He does not accept the fact that he is in the hospital. As you approach him, he makes the following comment.

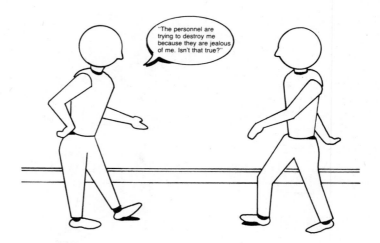

1. Give your immediate feeling response to the above situation.
2. Give your verbal and nonverbal response to the above situation.

Situation D. Mrs. Jeckel is a 42-year-old woman who sits in a chair all day and repeats over and over again how unworthy she is. You decide to sit with her. As you approach her, she makes the following comment:

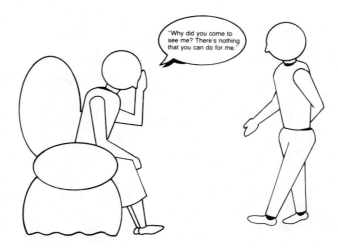

1. Give your immediate feeling response to the above situation.
2. Give your verbal and nonverbal response to the above situation.

Situation E. Mr. Barton is a 36-year-old salesman. He is always on the go, talking loudly and critically about what is going on. As you enter his room, Mr. Barton makes the following comment:

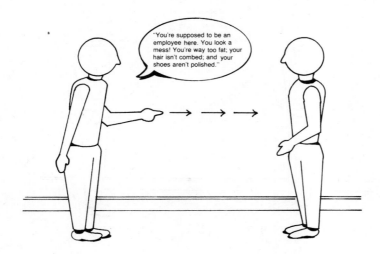

1. Give your immediate feeling response to the above situation.
2. Give your verbal and nonverbal response to the above situation.

Situation F. Mr. Tuttle is an 80-year-old man who is disoriented as to time and place. He has trouble finding his room and the bathroom and still thinks that he is back on the farm. As you approach him, he makes the following request:

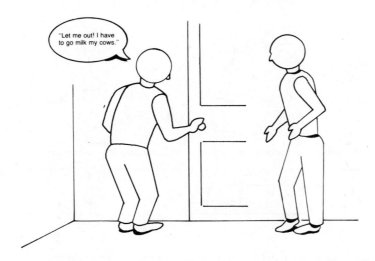

1. Give your immediate feeling response to the above situation.
2. Give your verbal and nonverbal response to the above situation.

Situation G. Mr. Felton is a 35-year-old man who has just been admitted for the twelfth time for alcoholism. While you are admitting him, he relates the following:

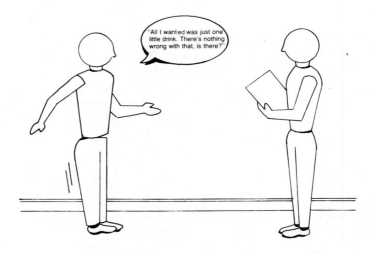

1. Give your immediate feeling response to the above situation.
2. Give your verbal and nonverbal response to the above situation.

Situation H. Molly McGee is a 38-year-old woman who is mentally retarded and emotionally disturbed. She sits in her rocking chair all day, cuddling her doll. As you approach her, you notice a large puddle under her chair.

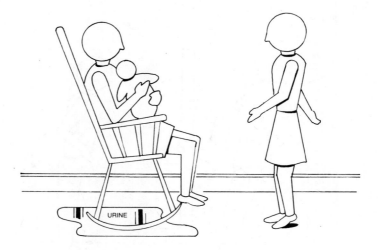

1. Give your immediate feeling response to the above situation.
2. Give your verbal and nonverbal response to the above situation.

Suggested Responses for Evaluation Exercise 1

SITUATION **A**

Responses should support reality and not focus on the client's complaints. For example: "I know at this time you probably feel you'll never get well. However, the symptoms are part of your illness. As you continue to work on your problem, your symptoms will gradually disappear."

SITUATION **B**

Responses should keep the client in contact with reality and offer direction, as necessary, to meeting activities of daily living. For example: "Mrs. Cannon, I'm Mrs. Troxel. It is time for dinner. I will walk with you to the dining room."

SITUATION **C**

Responses should neither agree nor disagree with client's ideas but should present reality in a matter-of-fact way. For example: "I can understand why you have this idea at this time, but this is not what is really going on."

SITUATION **D**

Responses should not support the client's negative view of self but should attempt to help the client function and focus outside of self. For example: "Perhaps there is nothing that I can do for you right now, but I would appreciate it if you could help me fold the laundry." (If the client follows through with this task, be sure to express your gratitude.)

SITUATION **E**

Responses should not be defensive, challenging, or retaliating but should indicate an attempt to constructively channel the client's overactivity. For example: "You might have a point there. It's a nice day. How about the two of us going for a walk?"

SITUATION **F**

Responses should reflect orientation to time, place, and person, and should utilize the client's past to orient him to the future. For example: "Mr. Tuttle, you are in the hospital now and not on the farm. But tell me about when you were a farmer and did your own milking. How early did you have to get up to start the milking?"

SITUATION **G**

Responses should be nonjudgmental. For example: "Obviously, Mr. Felton, you did not have just one drink for you to be admitted to the Mental Health Center."

SITUATION **H**

Responses should not reprimand the client but should include alternatives. For example: "Molly, you are wet. Let's go to your room and change your clothes." (Start Molly on a regular bathroom schedule. Take her to the bathroom every two hours.)

EVALUATION EXERCISE 2

THE PROBLEM-SOLVING PROCESS

STEPS	PROBLEM
1. Define the problem. What is actually causing the discomfort? (Sometimes this is difficult to pinpoint.)	
2. Decide on a goal.	
3. Identify alternatives. (There is always more than one way to solve a problem.)	
4. Choose an alternative.	
5. Try out the alternative.	
6. Evaluate the effectiveness.	
7. Repeat the process if the solution is not effective.	

EVALUATION EXERCISE 3

Health Provider's Interactions That Enhance the Client's Human Dignity and Worth

* Score yourself on the behaviors listed below.
* If you comply with any of the five positive behaviors, you are doing well.
* If you comply with four of the five positive behaviors, you are doing very well.
* If you comply with *all* of the five positive behaviors, you are enhancing the human value of *all* of your clients.

1. *Listening to what the patient has to say*
   For example: "You were telling me, Joe, about what you did on the weekend. I would like to hear more about what you did."
2. *Being consistent in the care that is given the patient*
   For example: Follow the plan of care that has been developed for the client. If you don't agree with the plan, bring it up at the care planning conference.
3. *Relating to adult clients as adults*
   For example: Use "I" messages, such as, "I would like you to. . ." instead of "You should . . . ."
4. *Focusing on the strengths of the client. Giving credit for positive behavior*
   For example: "You're going out to look for a job today; that's a good decision," or "You brushed your teeth by yourself; that's great."
5. *Recognizing the presence of the client unless this behavior, as specified in the plan of care, is not to be supported*
   For example: Client comes to the desk. Health provider acknowledges client by saying, "Is there something I can help you with?"

Scoring Sheet

ENHANCING BEHAVIORS	DAYS				
	1	2	3	4	5
1. Listening to what the client has to say					
2. Being consistent in the care that is given the client					
3. Relating to adult clients as adults					
4. Focusing on the *strengths* of the client. Giving credit for positive behavior					
5. Recognizing the presence of the client, unless this behavior is not to be supported					
	number of times				

EVALUATION EXERCISE 4

CROSSWORD PUZZLE

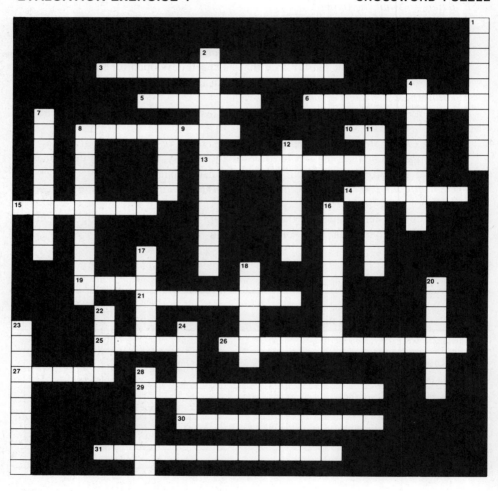

ACROSS

3. Transfer of feelings to a less threatening object
5. Original support group
6. Plusses in a person's life
8. Opposite of discipline
10. Abbreviation for delayed intellectual development
13. Undivided attention in conversation
14. Rejection of things as they actually are
15. Imaginary achievements
19. A biological, social or psychological hole in an individual's life
21. Prevention from reaching a goal
25. An antagonistic feeling
26. Exaggerating a desirable trait
27. An aspect of caring
29. Attitude or behavior when secure with oneself
30. Channeling anxiety into physical symptoms
31. Incorporation of another's standards so that they are not external threats

DOWN

1. Unconscious forcing of unpleasant experiences into the unconscious
2. Giving a logical sounding excuse that conceals the real reason
4. Attacking behavior in response to frustration and hostile feelings
7. Moving away from reality
8. Inpatient facility for care
9. A way of taking care of oneself
11. Retreating to earlier patterns of behavior
12. Activity to fulfill a need
16. Inner perceptions perceived as having origins outside of self
17. Negative actions cancelled out by other actions
18. Chemical coping
20. Specific plan of action
22. Measurable and attainable achievements
23. Morbid sadness
24. Physical impairment of the brain
28. Vague, uncomfortable feeling

Answers to Crossword Puzzle on next page

ANSWERS TO CROSSWORD PUZZLE

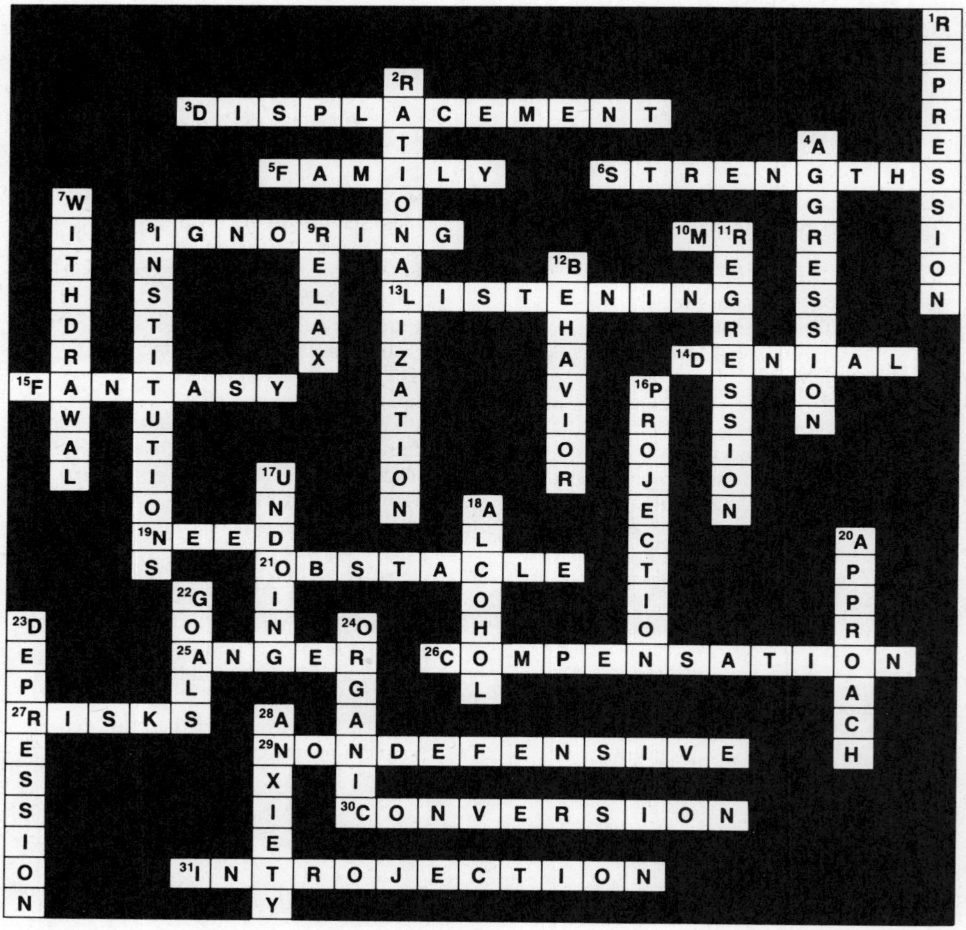
1 REPRESSION
2 RATIONALIZATION
3 DISPLACEMENT
4 AGGRESSION
5 FAMILY
6 STRENGTHS
7 WITHDRAWAL
8 IGNORING
8 INSTITUTIONS
9 RELAX
10 M
11 REGRESSION
12 BEHAVIOR
13 LISTENING
14 DENIAL
15 FANTASY
16 PROJECTION
17 UNDOING
18 ALCOHOL
19 NEED
20 APPROACH
21 OBSTACLE
22 GOALS
23 DEPRESSION
24 ORGANIC
25 ANGER
26 COMPENSATION
27 RISKS
28 ANXIETY
29 NONDEFENSIVE
30 CONVERSION
31 INTROJECTION

GLOSSARY

Acting out—socially unacceptable ways of expressing thoughts and feelings through behavior.

Addiction—a strong physical or emotional dependence on one thing, such as drugs, alcohol, running, eating, smoking. Depending on the purpose it serves, it can be positive or negative.

Additive effect—the combined effect of taking two drugs that is more than a 1 + 1 effect. For example, combining two central nervous system depressant drugs may affect the individual as though he had had multiple doses of the drugs. Overdose or death may result from this effect.

Adjustment—adapting to the demands of life.

Affect—pleasant or unpleasant feelings in response to an act or event.

Affective psychosis—a usually recurrent mental disorder characterized by a severe disturbance in mood.

Agitated—disturbed, upset, excited; apparent in the face or movements of the involved person.

Aggression—attacking behavior that occurs in response to frustration and hostile feelings.

Agranulocytosis—a blood dyscrasia characterized by decreased granulocytes and lesions of the throat and other mucous membranes, including the gastrointestinal tract and skin.

Akasthesia—an extrapyramidal side effect characterized by motor restlessness and anxiety even when at rest.

Alcoholism—chronic use of alcohol that ultimately interferes with health and activities of daily living.

Altered libido—change in sexual desire.

Ambivalence—existence of opposing emotions, such as love and hate, at the same time.

Anhidrosis—an abnormal deficiency or inability to sweat.

Antianxiety agent—medication that reduces anxiety and muscular tension.

Anticholinergic effects—autonomic side effects that include dry mouth, dysphagia, postural hypotension, urinary hesitancy or retention, constipation, and anhidrosis.

Antidepressive agent—medication used to treat depression.

Antimanic agent—lithium carbonate; specific to reducing symptoms of manic episodes and preventing recurrence of manic or depressive episodes.

Antipsychotic agent—medication used to decrease and control symptoms of psychotic disorders.

Anxiety—a feeling of impending doom accompanied by physical symptoms, such as diaphoresis, tachycardia, tremors, gastrointestinal symptoms.

Apathy—absence of feeling.

Applied behavioral analysis—systematic application of principles of behavior; also known as behavior modification and behavior management.

Assertiveness—a way of accepting responsibility for oneself by expressing thoughts and feelings directly and honestly without blaming self or others.

Assaultiveness—inflicting verbal or physical harm.

Ataxia—muscular coordination failure resulting in a staggering gait.

Attitude—the inclination to react positively or negatively to people or events.

Behavior—activity that can be observed.

Blood dyscrasias—an abnormal condition of the blood.

Blunting—dull or flat emotional response.

Blocking—sudden stoppage of thought, speech, or action for psychological reasons.

Body language—nonverbal communication of one's thoughts and feelings.

Burnout—a term coined to refer to the emotional exhaustion of the health provider.

Care plan (plan of care)—directions for individualizing client care. Problems are ordered and goals and approaches are specific to the problem stated. All goals are time-limited and measurable.

Catatonic motor behavior—reduction of spontaneous movement or excited motor activity, apparently purposeless and not influenced by external stimuli.

Client/patient/resident—individual receiving mental health services.

Commitment—decision by the court for involuntary treatment of a client for a limited amount of time, based on the client's dangerousness to self and others.

Communication—verbal and nonverbal means of conveying thoughts and feelings to others.

Compulsion—an undesired, repetitive action symbolic of unresolved problems; used to lower feelings of overwhelming anxiety.

Confabulation—making up stories to fill in memory gaps; seen especially in organic psychosis.

Confidentiality—client's right to privacy regarding details of his psychiatric care.

Contact dermatitis—a skin rash caused by direct contact between the skin and the allergic substance. Itching, blisters, oozing, and scaling are common symptoms.

Conversion—separating anxiety-producing problems from awareness by developing motor or sensory symptoms that symbolize the unresolved problem.

Coping—dealing with stress-producing situations in a positive or negative way.

Crisis—a sudden change of events that may create a potentially unbearably high level of stress for the individual.

Cue—a prompt or signal to get an individual's attention.

Data Base (baseline data)—number of times a behavior occurs before a program is implemented.

Defective judgment—inability to make wise decisions.

Defensive techniques—methods that are used to protect oneself without hurting the attacker.

Delirium tremens—tachycardia, diaphoresis, elevated blood pressure, due to withdrawal from heavy alcohol ingestion.

Delusion—belief or idea that is not supported by logic.

Dementia—loss of intellectual abilities, memory impairment, and other brain functions due to organic causes.

Denial—a coping/mental mechanism whereby the individual refuses to recognize the existence of a personal problem. A major coping mechanism of the alcoholic individual.

Depression—a disorder of mood characterized by sleep disturbance; change in appetite; weight gain or weight loss; decreased libido; loss of energy; fatigue; feelings of worthlessness; slowed thinking; and suicidal ideation.

Developmental stages—predictable, orderly levels of individual growth and development from birth to death.

Diagnosis—a way of categorizing disorders according to predetermined criteria for treatment, reporting, and compensation purposes.

Disorientation—inability to identify person, place, or time.

Displacement—unconscious coping/mental mechanism. Individual does not deal with source of frustration or anger directly, but takes it out on someone less threatening.

Distress—negative or uncomfortable stress; stress that overwhelms.

Drug abuse—misuse of prescribed or illicit drugs to attain an effect that is not considered appropriate.

Dry mouth—drug-induced effect on the mucous membranes in the mouth.

DSM III—Diagnostic Statistical Manual, third edition. A systematic way of classifying mental disorders.

Dysphagia—inability to swallow; may be drug-induced or caused by illness.

Dysphoric mood—feeling of anxiety, restlessness, or dissatisfaction.

Dystonia—an extrapyramidal side effect. Client experiences rigidity and spasms of the arms, legs, and neck muscles; has difficulty swallowing and speaking.

Ego—one of three major parts of personality, as described by Freud. Considered the moderator between the Id (primitive drive) and the Superego (conscience).

Electroconvulsive therapy—used to treat psychotic depression and break up compulsive suicidal ideation. A small amount of electrical current applied to head (brain) induces convulsions.

Emotion—strong feeling that influences behavior.

Emotional lability—sudden variations in mood, such as explosive temper outbursts and sudden crying.

Empathy—ability to understand what someone is feeling without experiencing the emotion oneself.

Extrapyramidal reaction—Parkinson-like actions including tremors, rigidity, drooling, mask-like facies, speech and writing difficulties, difficulty swallowing, gait disturbance, and pain and insomnia due to cramps and muscle spasm.

Fantasy—a coping/mental mechanism often likened to daydreaming.

Facial grimaces—contortions of the face due to physical or psychogenic reasons. May also be drug-induced.

Feedback—the part of communication that informs you that you have been understood.

Feelings of unreality—a sense of not existing or of being in a place other than where you are. Also called depersonalization.

Flatness of affect—lack of outward expression of feeling or emotion.

Flight of ideas—rapid switching from topic to topic. Ideas are complete as far as they go but are not finished. A common characteristic in manic disorders.

Functional disorder—mental disorder caused by overwhelming internal or external stressors.

Gastrointestinal disturbance—symptoms include nausea, vomiting, diarrhea, abdominal pain, and loss of appetite.

Grandiosity—unrealistic ideas about one's own significance or identity.

Group work—therapeutic, goal-directed activity for two or more clients with similar needs.

Guilt—a subjective feeling of self-blame regarding life experiences.

Hallucination—a false sensory perception that is real to the individual and not changed by logic.

Health provider—any mental health care worker who supervises or gives direct care to the client. For example, nurse, aide or orderly, psychiatrist, psychologist, social worker, activity therapist, recreation therapist, vocational therapist, behavioral analyst, alcoholism counselor, nutritionist, pharmacist.

Homicidal ideation—strong thoughts about the killing of one human being by another.

Hostility—antagonistic or angry feelings directed toward another.

Humanism—valuing the uniqueness, worth, and dignity of each individual.

Hyperactivity—above-normal increase in activity. May be due to physical or psychological causes.

Id—according to Freud, the primitive part of personality that operates on "I want what I want when I want it."

Ideas of persecution—beliefs, not based on reality, that someone is "out to get" the individual.

Ideas of reference—an individual's false interpretation that others' actions, conversations, or thoughts are about him.

Identification—a coping/mental mechanism especially common during adolescence. The individual thinks, feels, and acts like members of his peer group or a person significant to him.

Illusion—a misperception of reality. For example, perceiving a piece of lint as a bug.

Impulse—the urge to do something without considering the consequences.

Incoherence—loose, rambling, disjointed sentences.

Indifference to environment—lack of interest or concern in regard to what is going on around him.

Inhibition of ejaculation—a man's inability to release semen during intercourse. Can be drug-induced due to the autonomic (drying) effect or endocrine side effect.

Insight—understanding the reasons for one's own thoughts, feelings, and actions.

Insomnia—inability to sleep.

Introjection—a coping/mental mechanism in which the individual incorporates or internalizes conflicting values, standards, persons, objects, or attitudes so they are no longer an external threat.

Irrelevance—not applicable or pertinent.

Jaundice—a symptom caused by bilirubin in the blood and the depositing of bilirubin pigment, resulting in yellowness of the skin and white outer coat of the eyeballs, mucous membranes, and excretions.

Lactation—secretion of milk by the breast.

Lawful relationship (functional relationship)—relationship that establishes causes and effect; that is, a relationship in which some change in one event brings about corresponding change in a second event.

Loss of accommodation—inability of the muscles that control the lens of the eye to adjust for near or distant vision. May be the result of aging or drugs.

Mania—marked disturbance in mood characterized by increased activity, pressure to keep talking, flight of ideas, inflated self-esteem, decreased need for sleep, distractibility, or excessive involvement in impulsive, foolish behaviors.

Manipulation—influencing or arranging for one's own benefit.

Mental—referring to the mind.

Mental retardation—significant subaverage functioning, with IQ of 70 or below and onset before age 18.

Modeling—setting an example to follow.

Mood—emotion.

Motivation—the internal process that makes individuals behave as they do.

Motor retardation—abnormal decrease in motor activity. Common during severe depression. May also be caused by drugs or physical conditions.

Mutism—inability or refusal to speak.

Narcissism—self love; a common characteristic of the infant.

Negativism—resistance to doing what is expected or desirable.

Neologism—coining of new words that have meaning to the client but are not understood by others.

Neurosis—minor mental disorder characterized by free-floating anxiety. Unresolved problems are expressed somatically, through physical symptoms; or symbolically, through emotional symptoms.

Obsession—repetitive, unwanted idea that is symbolic of an unresolved problem or conflict.

Ocular changes—eye changes, such as loss of accommodation.

One-to-one relationship—therapeutic relationship between a client and health provider.

Organic mental illness—emotional illness due to physical impairment of the brain.

Panic—overwhelming anxiety that results in the individual's inability to function in an appropriate way.

Paradoxical behavior change—drug-induced; what the individual experiences is directly opposite to the expected effect of the drug (i.e., the drug increases the undesirable behavior). Often, this behavior is interpreted as part of the client's emotional illness.

Paranoid—pathological suspiciousness.

Pseudoparkinsonism—refers to drug-induced symptoms that mimic Parkinson's disease.

Personality—sum total of all that a person is.

Phobia—exaggeration of normal fear that creates panic when client is faced with that object or situation symbolic of unresolved problem or conflict.

Photosensitivity—individual develops redness of the exposed skin areas with intense burning or itching; may be drug-induced. Looks like severe case of sunburn.

Physical abuse—inflicting bodily injury on another.

Poor concentration—lack of ability to focus on the issue at hand.

Postural hypotension—lowering of blood pressure due to postural changes from lying or standing position. May cause momentary fainting and dizziness.

Premack principle (Grandma's rule)—first you must do what you don't really want to do before you can do something you like to do.

Pressure of speech—more talkativeness than usual with pressure to keep talking.

Problem—any question or situation that arises from a felt difficulty.

Problem-solving process—a systematic method of finding a solution to a question or situation that is a felt difficulty.

Projection—a coping/mental mechanism whereby an individual attributes his own weaknesses to others.

Psychiatry—a medical specialty that involves study, treatment, and prevention of mental illness.

Psychosis—major mental illness characterized by being out of touch with reality, inability to continue activities of daily living, disrupted interpersonal relationships, and lack of insight regarding the illness. There is overall severe interference in thinking, feeling, and doing.

Psychotherapy—sometimes referred to as talk therapy. Deals with emotional problems, either individually or in a group, with a psychotherapist.

Rationalization—a coping/mental mechanism in which the individual offers a logical, but untrue reason as an excuse for his behavior.

Reality—that which is true and actually exists.

Regression—a coping/mental mechanism during which the individual reverts to behavior characteristic of a less stressful time of life.

Replacement—term used by placement specialists who deal directly with the mentally ill population. It refers to the client who worked prior to hospitalization and now has been reintroduced into a vocational setting.

Resistiveness—opposition to what is suggested or desired by others.

Schizophrenia—a group of psychotic disorders characterized by severe interference in thinking, feeling, and doing. According to DSM-III, one must have continuous signs of the illness for at least six months for a diagnosis of schizophrenia.

Sedation—common side effect of many psychotherapeutic medications. A quieting, calming effect. Individual may have eyes closed but is not asleep. Will usually respond to conversation with single words.

Skin disorders—includes allergic reactions, such as itching, redness, rash, and hives.

Skin pigmentation—drug-induced discoloration of the skin ranging from a darkening to a slate gray to a violet hue. Generally restricted to exposed areas; rare.

Social withdrawal—seclusiveness.

Somatic concern—preoccupation with physical illness or bodily functions, such as constipation.

Stimulus—object or event.

Stress—psychological and physical response to real or imagined pressure.

Sublimation—a positive coping/mental mechanism in which the individual converts potentially negative drives into positive action.

Suicidal tendencies—individual has either attempted suicide or has a strong desire to do so.

Suicide—to deliberately take one's own life.

Superego—according to Freud, that part of personality that acts as the censoring agent or conscience.

Symbolization—a coping/mental mechanism that represents an internal feeling, wish, attitude, or idea through an external object or quality.

Sympathy—a common response in personal relationships where an individual experiences the friend's feeling or mood.

Synapse—a fluid-filled space between the neurons.

Tachycardia—abnormally rapid heart rate.

Tardive dyskinesia—a late-occurring side effect of antipsychotic medication that is probably permanent; results in involuntary repetitive movements of the face, cheek, mouth, and neck muscles.

Thought disorganization—absence of orderly organization of thinking.

Uncooperativeness—an unwillingness or lack of ability to work together.

Uncommunicativeness—since persons communicate nonverbally, as well as verbally, this term is limited to lack of verbal communication.

Unusual thought content—thinking is different from that accepted as normal by society. Delusions are an example of unusual thought content.

Urticaria—hives; red or pale raised patches on the skin often accompanied by severe itching.

Values clarification—making personal values clear to oneself.

Withdrawal from reality—functioning within one's own created reality that is not a part of the real world.

INDEX